NEUROSCIENCE RESEARCH PROGRESS

DUAL PROCESSING MODEL OF VISUAL INFORMATION: CORTICAL AND SUBCORTICAL PROCESSING

NEUROSCIENCE RESEARCH PROGRESS

NEUROSCIENCE RESEARCH PROGRESS

DUAL PROCESSING MODEL OF VISUAL INFORMATION: CORTICAL AND SUBCORTICAL PROCESSING

HITOSHI SASAKI

Nova Science Publishers, Inc.
New York

LIBRARY OF CONGRESS CATALOGING-IN-PUBLICATION DATA

Sasaki, Hitoshi, Ph. D.
 Dual processing model of visual information : cortical and subcortical processing / Hitoshi Sasaki.
    p. ; cm.
 Includes bibliographical references and index.
 ISBN 978-1-60876-399-3 (softcover)
 1. Visual cortex. 2. Visual perception. I. Title.
 [DNLM: 1. Visual Perception--physiology. 2. Dominance, Cerebral. 3. Visual Cortex--physiology. WW 105 S252d 2009]
 QP383.15.S27 2009
 612.8'255--dc22
                            2009039003

Published by Nova Science Publishers, Inc. ✛ *New York*

CONTENTS

PREFACE

In order to investigate a possible role of visual processing in the regulation of adaptive behaviors, two behavioral experiments using color stimulus were performed in human subjects. In the first experiment, hemispheric asymmetry of color processing was investigated by measuring reaction time to a stimulus presented either in the left or the right visual field responded by the ipsilateral hand. The simple reaction time was shorter to a color stimulus presented in the right hemisphere in the right-handed participants, while no hemispheric asymmetry was found in color discrimination reaction time without verbal cues. In the second experiment, a modulatory effect of color on sensorimotor gating was investigated using a prepulse inhibition task. Amplitude of a startle-eyeblink response elicited by an air-puff to the cornea was significantly inhibited by a shortly (100 ms) preceding color prepulse. Different color prepulses induced different degrees of the inhibition. A yellow prepulse was more effective as compared to a blue one. Although the exact neuronal pathways underlying the prepulse inhibition of the corneal blink response remain to be determined, a top-down pathway from the cortex to the brainstem nuclei via the amygdala seems to be involved in the sensorimotor gating. From these findings combined with other studies, I propose here a dual-processing hypothesis of visual inputs, where physical features of the stimulus are processed in the cerebral cortex with consciousness, while the psychological and biological meanings are processed mainly in the limbic system without consciousness. Traditionally, it was thought that these two processes are in series, while in the present model these processes are in parallel, in addition to the serial processing. Visual inputs are conveyed to the limbic system via the indirect cortical and the direct subcortical pathways. The cortical pathway further divided into two routs; one is from the inferotemporal cortex and the other is from the posterior parietal association cortex through the pulvinar nucleus of the thalamus. The subcortical pathway diverges from the extrageniculostriatal visual pathway at the posterior thalamus.

Chapter 1

INTRODUCTION

Color is one of attributes of an object. However, color does not belong to the object itself, but is produced in the organism that receives it. Indeed, sight of mono- or dichromatic observers is so different from normal trichromatic sight. It is well known that only a black and white stimulus can produce color sensation if it is presented in a certain spatio-temporal arrangement. Benham's top (see review by von Campenhausen and Schramme, 1995) is a famous example showing that color does not belong to the physical object itself, but depends on physiological and psychological events, which are produced in the visual system (Newton, 1672).

Color processing is a function of the visual cortex (Zeki et al,, 1991; Corbetta et al., 1991; De Valois and De Valois, 1993; Ungerleider and Haxby, 1994). However, little is known about the hemispheric difference of the color processing. Moreover, there are a few studies, which examined functional meanings of color information. In the present chapter, two experiments will be described to answer these questions; one examines the hemispheric asymmetry of color processing, and the other examines the effect of color on modulating a startle reflex in normal human subjects.

Results of these experiments will clearly demonstrate that the right hemisphere superiority in color detection in right-handed participants, and that color information modulates the startle reflex by a subcortical pathway to the brain stem, presumably via the limbic system. From these results and related findings, I propose a new hypothesis that the sensory inputs, in general, are analyzed and processed in two evolutionary different systems (limbic and neocortex) to elicit adaptive behaviors to maintain homeostasis of the organism. A visual stimulus, including color, is processed in two systems in parallel; one is a modality-specific visual system and the other is a non-specific limbic system. Detailed, local physical features of the stimulus are processed in the former system with consciousness, while the global psychological and biological meanings are processed mainly in the latter system without consciousness.

These two systems are in parallel in nature with some interactions, and the outputs of the former system are transferred to the latter system.

Chapter 2

EXPERIMENT 1: HEMISPHERIC ASYMMETRY IN COLOR PROCESSING

2.1. Background

2.1.1. Anatomical Asymmetry of Brain

Bilateral asymmetries have been found in the human brain; they tend to be larger right than left prefrontal and larger left than right occipital lobe volume (Foundas et al., 2003). Asymmetry has been also reported in several subcortical structures. Amygdalar and hippocampal volume measurements indicate a right-greater-than-left asymmetry for right-handed normal participants (Jack et al., 1989; Szabo et al., 2001). These structural asymmetries suggest functional lateralization of various cerebral functions.

2.1.2. Hemispheric Lateralization of Cerebral Functions

It has been suggested that the left hemisphere plays an important role in linguistic and higher order cognitive processes, such as self-recognition (McFie et al., 1950; Conway et al., 1999; Turk et al., 2002), whereas the right hemisphere is responsible for visuospatial perception and facial recognition (Kimura, 1969; Gazzaniga and LeDoux, 1978; Sergent et al., 1992; Haxby et al., 1994; Kanwisher et al., 1997; Barton et al., 2002; Corballis, 2003).

Several researchers have postulated lateralized function regarding each hemisphere. The right-hemisphere functions were referred to as "visuospatial," or "constructional" (Sperry, 1982). It has also been suggested that the right hemisphere is specialized for the analysis of global-level information, and serves as an anomaly detector, while the left hemisphere tends to create a "story" to make sense of the incongruities (Ramachandran and Blakeslee, 1998; Smith et al, 2002). Levy (1969) studied an organizational differentiation of the hemispheres for perceptual and cognitive functions and supposed that the left hemisphere is specialized for analytic processing and the right hemisphere is specialized for integrative processing. In addition, the left hemisphere is specific in logical processing, while the right one has superiority in emotion, music, and holistic processing (Levy, 1969; Ladavas et al., 1984; Magnani et al., 1984; Patel et al., 1998). Little is known, however, about hemispheric asymmetry in color processing. In the first experiment, we examined the hemispheric lateralization of color processing.

2.1.3. Hemispheric Asymmetry Using Reaction Time

Lateralized function in the cerebral hemisphere has been studied by using several methods, such as a same-different comparison task (Hannay, 1979), a list-learning procedure (Berry, 1990), tachistoscopic presentation (Malone and Hannay, 1978), and reaction time (Davidoff, 1976). These different methods reveal the different features of the cerebral function. However, the input information presented to either one of the hemispheres immediately transfers to the other hemisphere via the commisure fibers. The interhemispheric transfer time is estimated from 2 to 6 ms (Poffenberger, 1912; Berlucchi et al., 1971; Brizzolara et al., 1994; Brysbaert, 1994). Therefore, in order to detect a difference in the processing time between two hemispheres, a method with high time resolution should be used. The reaction time task has an advantage that it is sensitive to analyze the differences in time for information processing in the hemispheres.

2.1.4. Reaction Time Task Based Upon Double-Crossed Projections

The optic nerve fibers originating from the nasal retina project to the contralateral visual cortex, while the others from the temporal retina project to the ipsilateral visual cortex, and the right motor cortex innervates the left hand and the left one innervates the right hand. Hemispheric dominance in color processing can be evaluated by using a reaction time task based upon these double-crossed projections of the visual and pyramidal pathway features in human participants (Poffenberger, 1912; Berlucchi et al., 1971).

2.2. Experiment 1-1: Reaction Time Difference by the Dominant and the Non-Dominant Hands

2.2.1. Purpose

Hemispheric asymmetry can be evaluated based on the difference in reaction times to lateralized stimuli presented either in the left or the right visual field and responded to by the ipsilateral hand (Fig.1). The first experiment was designed to evaluate a difference of reaction times between the dominant and non-dominant hands using achromatic targets presented at the center of the visual field. The results of this experiment will serve as a control for difference of reaction time by different hands.

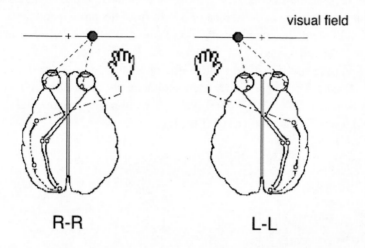

Figure 1. Schematic representation of experimental conditions used in the Experiment 1. Reaction time was measured to a target presented in the right visual field by the right hand (R-R, the left hemisphere) or the left visual field by the left hand (L-L, the right hemisphere).

2.2.2. Methods

2.2.2.1. Participants

Ten right-handed undergraduate students (3 males and 7 females) with normal or corrected normal vision (mean age 19.5 years, SD 2.7) participated in the first experiment. Most of the participants were selected from ten groups consisting of eight subjects in a preliminary experiment because they showed the smallest variability and the shortest reaction time in each group. In the preliminary experiment, thirteen simple reaction times to color stimuli (either red, green, blue, or yellow) presented at the center of a cathode ray tube (CRT) display were recorded. No 'ready' signal was used in the preliminary experiment. All the participants were naive to this kind of behavioral experiment and the experiments were performed with the consent of each participant.

2.2.2.2. Apparatus

An achromatic solid circle with a diameter of 2 deg (x = 0.283, y = 0.320, CIE) was presented on a CRT display (Panasonic TX-D7P35-J, Japan, with a resolution of 800 x 600 dots at 60 Hz, 9300K). The luminous intensity of the target was 12, 14, or 18 cd/m^2 with a uniform gray background of 10 cd/m^2. The CRT display was placed at a distance of 57 cm from the participant's eye. All the visual stimuli were generated using a graphic generator (VSG Series Three, Cambridge Research Systems Ltd., England).

Reaction time was measured using a programmable logic controller (Keyence KV24AT, Japan). The experiments were automatically controlled by a computer (Power Macintosh 7300/180, Apple), using a hand-made program (HyperCard, Apple) and a serial/parallel interface (Fig. 2).

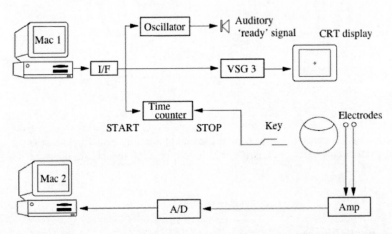

Figure 2. Schematic illustration of experimental set-up for the reaction time to visual stimulus. Presentation of an auditory 'ready' signal, target visual stimuli and trigger of a time counter was controlled by a computer (Mac 1) via an interface unit (I/F). The visual stimuli were generated by a graphic generator (VSG 3) and were presented on a CRT display. Reaction time was measured by the time counter. EOG signals were amplified (Amp) and stored in another computer (Mac 2) after digitized (A/D) at 400 Hz.

Electro-oculogram (EOG) was recorded from two small electrodes with a diameter of 5 mm placed 2 cm above or below the lateral edges of right and left eyes. The signal was amplified with a time constant of 1.5 sec and a high-cut filter at 60 Hz (Nihon Kohden, EEG-4316, Japan), and was recorded on a computer (Power Macintosh 7100/80AV, Apple) after being digitized at 400 Hz (MacLab, AD Instruments, Australia). If the amplitude of EOG exceeded 50 μV, which corresponded to an eye-movement of 3 deg in the visual angle, or if an eye blink occurred at the time of stimulus presentation, the trial was omitted from later analysis. In addition, trials with reaction times longer than 400 ms were omitted from later analysis. Thus, about 10 % of the trials were omitted as error trials.

2.2.2.3. Procedures

Participants were seated in a sound-attenuated chamber, facing the CRT display. Each participant's head was loosely restrained by using a chin rest, and the participant was asked to fixate at a small cross (0.5 deg, 0.5 deg) presented at the center of the CRT display. An auditory 'ready' signal preceded the onset of the target stimulus by 1-4 sec (mean 2.5 sec), and the delays were delivered in a quasi-random order (Fig. 3).

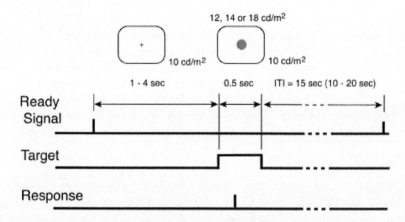

Figure 3. Schematic illustration of a time schedule for Experiment 1-1. A trial started with an auditory 'ready' signal preceding 1-4 sec with a mean of 2.5 sec. A target was presented for 0.5 sec at the center of the CRT display, where a small cross was presented as a fixation point. A total of 15 trials were performed with an inter-trial interval of 10-20 sec with a mean of 15 sec. The target was a gray circle with a diameter of 2 deg at either12, 14 or 18 cd/m² with a gray background of 10 cd/m².

Two blocks of experiments were performed with an inter-block interval of about 5 min. In each block, participants were required to press the key as quickly as possible to each stimulus presented at the center of visual field (Fig. 4). Before starting each block, participants were instructed which hand to use and the order of hands used were randomized among the participants. Each block consisted of 15 trials with a randomized inter-trial interval of 15 sec ranging from 10 sec to 20 sec. The median reaction time was calculated for each block for each participant. The mean value was then obtained for each condition (right or left hand).

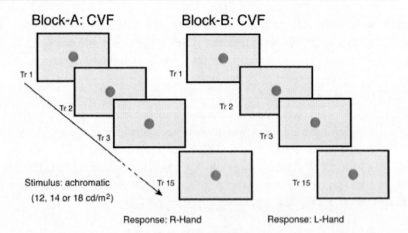

Figure. 4. Schematic drawing of procedure for Experiment 1-1. Two blocks, each consisting of 15 trials, were performed, using three different luminance stimuli (12, 14 or 18 cd/m^2) each with 5 trials. For both block-A and block-B, target was presented at the center of visual field (CVF). Response was made by the right hand (R-Hand) for block-A, and by the left hand (L-Hand) for block-B, respectively. Order of the blocks was randomized for each individual. Which block was performed had been informed before starting each block.

2.2.3. Results

There was no significant difference between the reaction times to achromatic stimulus presented at the center of visual field, and responded to by the dominant (right) and non-dominant (left) hands (Fig. 5). Figure 6 shows reaction times by the dominant and non-dominant hands to three different target luminances (12, 14 and 18 cd/m^2). Reaction time decreased gradually as a function of stimulus intensity. For both dominant and non-dominant hands, however, there was no significant difference between the reaction times of the right and left hands in any luminance condition. Statistical analysis using analysis of variance (ANOVA) showed that only the effect of luminance was significant ($F_{(2,18)} = 5.854$, $p < 0.01$), and both the effect of hands and the interaction between these two factors were not significant ($F_{(1,9)} = 0.019$, N.S., $F_{(2,18)} = 0.550$, N.S., respectively).

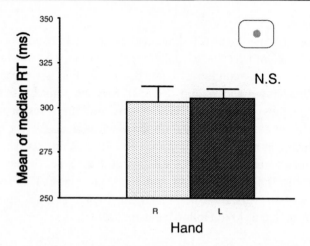

Figure 5. Simple reaction time by right (R, dominant) or left (L, non-dominant) hand to achromatic targets presented at the center of visual field in 10 right-handed participants. There was no significant (N.S.) difference between reaction times by dominant and non-dominant hands. Mean with SE.

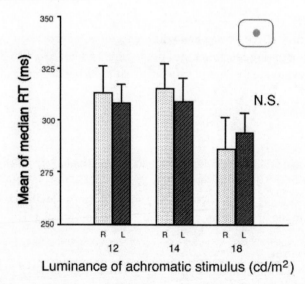

Figure 6. Simple reaction time by the right hand (R, dominant) or the left hand (L, non-dominant) to achromatic stimuli presented at the center of visual field in 10 right-handed participants. Means of median reaction time (mean with SE) were plotted against luminance of stimulus. Reaction times decreased with increase in luminance of stimulus. However, there was no significant (N.S.) difference between reaction times by dominant and non-dominant hands to visual stimuli in each luminance level (12, 14, and 18 cd/m^2).

2.2.4. Discussion

The results of Experiment 1-1 show that the dominant hand has no advantage over the non-dominant hand for the simple reaction time task, in which triggering simple hand-movement-initiation is required. This finding is well-consistent with previous studies (Hayes and Halpin, 1978; Annett and Annett, 1979; Adam and Vegge, 1991), thus confirming the validity of the present experimental procedures. The time required for the response selection and/or the motor control processes, which can be assumed to exist between stimulus presentation and the response (Schmidt and Lee, 1998), was suggested to be similar between the reaction times by the dominant and non-dominant hands. This means that no correction procedure is required when comparing reaction times by the dominant and non-dominant hands in the following experiments.

2.3. Experiment 1-2: Hemispheric Asymmetry of Color Detection in Right-Handed Subjects

2.3.1. Purpose

In this experiment, the hemispheric difference of color processing was evaluated by comparing reaction times of the right and left hands to chromatic stimuli presented to the ipsilateral visual field of right-handed individuals.

2.3.2. Materials and Methods

2.3.2.1. Participants

Ten right-handed undergraduate students (7 males and 3 females) with normal or corrected-to-normal vision (mean age 22.6 years, SD 6.1) participated in this experiment. All of these participants were selected from ten groups consisting of eight subjects in the preliminary experiment as in Experiment 1-1.

2.3.2.2. Apparatus

One of three chromatic solid circles with a diameter of 2 deg (red, $x = 0.553$, $y = 0.313$, CIE; green, $x = 0.279$, $y = 0.577$, CIE; or blue, $x = 0.226$, $y = 0.151$, CIE) was presented on the CRT display with a uniform gray background of 10 cd/m^2. All of these chromatic stimuli had the same saturation of 60%. The luminances of the chromatic stimuli were adjusted to a gray of 10 cd/m^2 using the flicker-photometry method so that it was equal for all participants, thus only the hue change served as a cue for the detection of the stimuli.

2.3.2.3. Procedures

Two blocks, each consisting of 15 trials, were performed, with an inter-block interval of about 5 min (Fig. 7, 8). For each block, participants were asked to press the key either by their right hands for targets presented in the right visual field (R-R condition), or by their left hands for targets in the left visual field (L-L condition). Before starting each block, the participants were told which hand to use, and on which side the stimuli will appear. Thus, there was no spatial cue for the response. The order of the blocks was randomized among participants. In each trial, one of the three chromatic targets was presented at 4 deg horizontally from the fixation point in either the right or left visual field (Fig. 8). The rest of the procedure was the same as in Experiment 1-1.

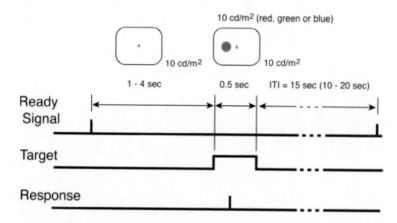

Figure 7. Schematic illustration of a time schedule for Experiment 1-2. A trial started with an auditory 'ready' signal preceding 1-4 sec with a mean of 2.5 sec. A target was presented at 4 deg lateral to the fixation point, either in the left or right visual field for 0.5 sec. A total of 15 trials were performed with an inter-trial interval of 10-20 sec with a mean of 15 sec. The target was a 2-deg chromatic circle of either red, green, or blue presented on a gray background of 10 cd/m^2.

2.3.3. Results

Figure 9 shows the reaction times to the chromatic targets in R-R and L-L conditions. In the right-handed participants, a mean reaction time in L-L (320±9 ms, mean ± SE) was shorter than that in R-R (303±9 ms, mean ± SE). Since there was no significant difference between reaction times to the target colors (red, green, and blue), the data was collapsed across cued color. A statistically significant difference was observed between reaction times in L-L and R-R (time difference was 17 ms, $t(9) = 3.171$, $p < 0.05$). The significant difference was still apparent if the analysis included only six right-handed participants who participated in both Experiments 1-2 and 1-4, in which lateralized achromatic stimuli were used for targets (t(5)=6.544, p < 0.01). Shorter reaction time in L-L was consistently observed in each of the three colors. These findings suggest that the right hemisphere is dominant in the detection of chromatic stimulus among right-handed participants.

2.3.4. Discussion

Clear, right hemisphere dominance in color detection was observed among the right-handed individuals. Difference of time in the color detection between the right hemisphere and the left hemisphere was 17 ms. This time-difference cannot be ascribed to the difference of hands, or motor process because there was no significant difference between reaction times by the dominant and non-dominant hands (Experiment 1-1). Thus, the time-difference should be ascribed to the difference in the processing of visual stimuli.

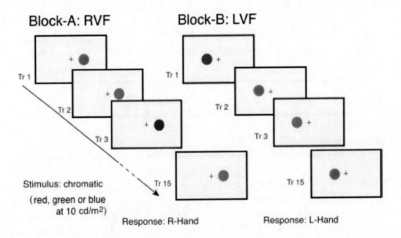

Figure 8. Schematic drawing of the procedure for Experiment 1-2. Two blocks, each consisting of 15 trials, were performed, using three different chromatic stimuli (red, green, or blue) each for 5 trials. For block-A, target was presented in the right visual field (RVF), and for block-B in the left visual field (LVF). Response was made by the right hand (R-Hand) for block-A, and by the left hand (L-Hand) for block-B, respectively. Order of the chromatic stimuli and of the blocks was randomized for each individual. Which block was tested had been informed before starting each block.

In the present study, we found hemispheric asymmetry in the detection of chromatic stimuli in normal subjects, not in patients. Present findings seem to be in good harmony with previous results, in which color discrimination is specialized for the right hemisphere (Davidoff, 1976; Pennal, 1977). However, in these prior studies, the target color stimuli were presented on a dark background of different luminances. Therefore, the appearance of the target was inevitably accompanied by a change in luminance, in addition to a change in hue. As it has been known that the salience of stimulus is one of the important variables that affect reaction time (Schmidt and Lee, 1998), if more than two attributes of a stimulus change simultaneously, the more salient attribute may overshadow the effects of the other (Sutherland and Mackintosh, 1971; Rescorla and Wagner, f1972; see Christman, 1989). In contrast, in the present study, we used color stimuli with the subjectively-equated luminance as the background to control all attributes as equal, except for hue.

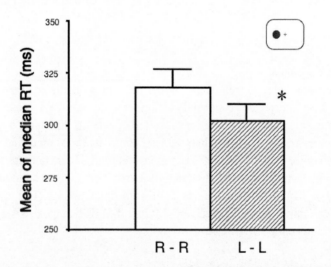

Figure 9. Simple reaction times by the right hand to chromatic targets presented in the right visual field (R-R), and by the left hand to targets presented in the left visual field (L-L) in 10 right-handed participants. Mean of median reaction time in L-L was significantly faster than in R-R (* p<0.05). Mean with SE. Insert is a schematic sample of stimulus presented in the left visual field.

Consistent with the present results, it has been reported that deficits in color detection in the contralateral visual field are more frequently observed in patients with a lesion of the right postero-occipital cerebral areas than the left ones (Scotti and Spinnler, 1970). Cortical color blindness has been also reported in patients with impairment of the left visual field (Albert et al., 1975). These findings imply that the right hemisphere is dominant in the detection of color among the right-handed individuals. However, to elucidate the neural mechanisms underlying the asymmetric processing in color detection, further studies should be done including recording of cortical activity during color detection task, and using methods with high time resolution.

2.4. Experiment 1-3: Hemispheric Asymmetry of Color Detection in Left-Handed Subjects

2.4.1. Purpose

In this experiment, the hemispheric difference of color processing was evaluated by comparing reaction times of the right and left hands to chromatic stimuli presented to the ipsilateral visual field of left-handed individuals.

2.4.2. Methods

2.4.2.1. Participants

Eight left-handed male subjects (7 undergraduate students and one researcher) with normal or corrected-to-normal vision (mean age 25.1 years, SD 9.3) participated in this experiment. All of these left-handed participants were selected based on an assessment of the handedness score using a modified Edinburgh Laterality Inventory (Oldfield, 1971), which included 7 items: write, eat, throw, tooth-brushing, drive, key, and hammer. For each item, right-handed responses were scored as 0, left-handed ones as 1, or both hands as 0.5. The total score of the left-handed participants ranged from 2.0 to 7.0 (4.6±1.6, mean ±SD), while the score of the right-handed participants was 0.

2.4.2.2. Apparatus and Procedures

The experimental apparatus and procedures for this experiment were similar for the Experiment 1-1 and 1-2, except that color stimuli were used to examine the effect of the dominant hand on the simple reaction time.

2.4.3. Results

Figure 10 shows that there was no significant difference between the simple reaction times by dominant and non-dominant hands in the left-handed participants.

There was no significant difference between simple reaction times to lateralized chromatic stimuli in R-R and L-L conditions among the left-handed participants (Fig. 11 left, R-R 325±5 ms, mean ± SE; L-L 324±9 ms, mean ± SE; t(7) = 0.179, N.S.). However, it might be assumed that the right hemisphere is more specialized in color detection among the left-handed individuals with a low left-handedness score, while symmetrical processing occurs among the typical left-handers with a high score. In order to ascertain this possibility, we performed the correlation analysis. No significant correlation between the handedness scores and reaction time differences (R-R − L-L) was observed (r = 0.006, p = 0.990, N.S.).

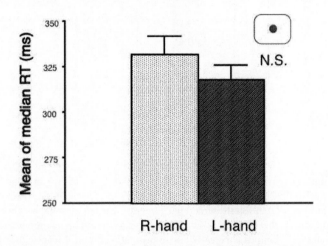

Figure 10. Simple reaction times to chromatic stimuli presented at the center of visual field, responded by the right hand (R-hand, non-dominant) and the left hand (L-hand, dominant) in 8 left-handed participants. There was no significant difference between reaction times by dominant and non-dominant hands. Mean with SE. Insert shows a schematic sample of stimulus presented at the center of visual field.

2.4.4. Discussion

A more symmetrical hemispheric processing was observed among left-handed individuals compared to right-handed individuals. It is well-known that language cerebral dominance is lateralized in the left hemisphere in 88-96% of right-handed individuals and in 43-76% of left-handers (Pujol et al., 1999; Springer et al., 1999; Khedr et al., 2002). It has been suggested that the hemispheric specialization of brain functions is less clear among left-handers than among right-handers (Zangwill, 1962, Bryden, 1982). Consistent with this concept, the present study showed that color detection was less clearly lateralized among the left-handed participants than among the right-handed participants

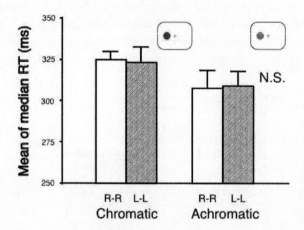

Figure 11. Simple reaction times to lateralized stimuli, responded by the right hand to targets presented in the right visual field (R-R), and by the left hand to targets presented in the left visual field (L-L) in 8 left-handed participants. Target stimulus was chromatic (left) or achromatic (right, 20 cd/m^2). There was no significant difference between reaction times in R-R and L-L, both to chromatic and achromatic stimuli. Mean with SE. Inserts are schematic samples of chromatic (left) and achromatic (right) stimuli presented in the left visual field.

2.5. Experiment 1-4: Hemispheric Asymmetry of Non-Color Detection in Right- and Left-Handed Subjects

2.5.1. Purpose

This experiment was designed to identify the critical factor for the asymmetry observed in Experiment 1-2. We determined whether the asymmetry observed in the detection of color might also be found in the detection of achromatic stimuli or not. If the asymmetry was lost using achromatic stimuli, it should therefore be ascribed to color processing and not to other factors.

2.5.2. Methods

2.5.2.1. Participants

Twelve right-handed (6 males and 6 females, mean age 20.5 years, SD 2.8) and eight left-handed undergraduate students participated in the present experiment. The six right-handed subjects were the same individuals who participated in Experiment 1-1, while the other six subjects were those who participated in Experiment 1-2. All left-handed subjects were those who participated in Experiment 1-3.

2.5.2.2. Apparatus

An achromatic, solid circle with a diameter of 2 deg (x = 0.283, y = 0.320, CIE) was presented on the CRT display with a uniform gray background of 10 cd/m² (Fig. 12). In the six right-handed participants who participated in Experiment 1-1, luminances of either 12, 14, or 18 cd/m² were tested, while in other six right-handed participants who participated in Experiment 1-2, as well as in the eight left-handed participants, only a luminance of 20 cd/m² was used.

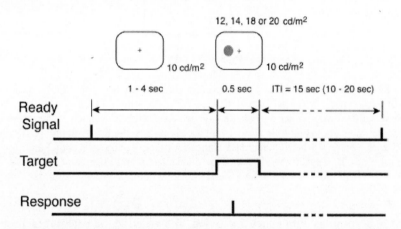

Figure 12. Schematic illustration of a time schedule for Experiment 1-4. A trial started with an auditory 'ready' signal preceding 1-4 sec with a mean of 2.5 sec. A target was presented at 4 deg lateral to the fixation point, either left or right visual field for 0.5 sec. A total of 15 trials were performed with an inter-trial interval of 10-20 sec with a mean of 15 sec. The target was an achromatic circle (x = 0.283, y = 0.320, CIE) with a diameter of 2 deg, either12, 14, 18 or 20 cd/m² with a gray background of 10 cd/m².

2.5.2.3. Procedures

The reaction times to achromatic stimuli presented in either the right hemisphere or the left hemisphere were recorded. In each block, the achromatic target was presented either on the right or the left visual field, at 4 deg horizontally from the fixation point (Fig. 13). Other experimental settings and procedures were the same as in Experiment 1-2.

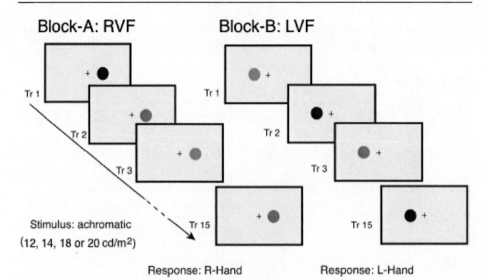

Figure 13. Schematic drawing of a procedure for Experiment 1-4. Two blocks, each consisting of 15 trials, were performed, using achromatic stimuli (12, 14 or 18 cd/m^2 in 6 participants, 20 cd/m^2 in other 6 participants) each for 5 trials. For block-A, target was presented in the right visual field (RVF), and for block-B in the left visual field (LVF). Response was made by the right hand (R-Hand) for block-A, and by the left hand (L-Hand) for block-B, respectively. Order of the blocks and stimuli were randomized for each individual. Which block was tested had been informed before starting each block.

2.5.3. Results

As the stimulus luminance increased, the reaction time to the achromatic stimulus decreased in the right-handed participants (Fig. 14). There was a statistically significant difference between the mean reaction time of 12, 14, or 18 cd/m^2 (N = 6) and the mean reaction time at 20 cd/m^2 (N = 12), in R-R and L-L conditions (t(10) = 3.221, p < 0.01; t(10) = 2.686, p < 0.05, respectively). However, at any target luminance, no significant difference was found between the reaction times to the achromatic stimuli among the right-handed participants in RR and LL conditions (W12, t(5) = 0.697, N.S.; W14, t(5) = 0.188, N.S.; W18, t(5) = 1.057, N.S.; W20, t(5) = 0.464, N.S.), even after this data was pooled (t(23) = 0.704, N.S.). Similarly, there was no significant difference between the reaction times to the achromatic stimuli among the eight left-handed participants in R-R and L-L conditions (308±11 ms, mean ± SE; 309±9 ms, mean ± SE, respectively; t(7) = 0.192, N.S., Fig. 11 right).

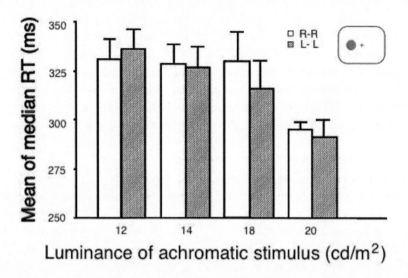

Luminance of achromatic stimulus (cd/m²)

Figure 14. Simple reaction times to achromatic stimuli presented either in the right visual field, responded by the right hand (R-R; open bars) and the left visual field by the left hand (L-L; hatched bars) in right-handed participants (n=6; 12, 14 or 18 cd/m², n=12; 20 cd/m²). The reaction time decreased as the stimulus luminance increased. In any case, however, there was no significant difference between reaction times in R-R and L-L. Mean with SE. Insert shows a schematic sample of stimulus presented in the left visual field.

2.5.4. Discussion

2.5.4.1 Effect of Luminance on Hemispheric Asymmetry

The decrement of reaction time with increasing luminance of target stimulus observed in Experiment 1-4 is well-consistent with previous reports. It has been known that reaction time depends on the intensity or salience of the stimulus (Lit et al., 1971; Jaskowski, 1982; Adams and Mamassian, 2004).

Although there are numerous studies investigating hemispheric asymmetry of luminance processing, only a few studies have explicitly examined the effects of stimulus luminance (see review by Christman, 1989). Christman (1990) varied luminances within a temporal integration task involving the identification of digits and found that increases in luminance tend to preferentially benefit the left hemisphere. Sergent (1982) varied luminances in a task requiring subjects to judge the gender of laterally-presented faces and found a shorter reaction time in the right hemisphere for low luminance (0.8 mL) and in the left hemisphere for high luminance stimuli (12.0 mL). More recently, Corballis et al. (2002) found in split-brain patients that luminance discrimination was processed equivalently by the two hemispheres. Thus, there is no general consensus regarding whether there is hemispheric asymmetry in the detection speed of the achromatic patch stimulus used in the present study. Since we have used chromatic stimuli with constant luminance (Experiment 1-2), luminance itself does not seem to be an important factor for a right hemisphere advantage found in Experiment 1-2. No significant asymmetry was observed in the luminance-detection task in Experiment 1-4. Therefore, the asymmetry obtained in Experiment 1-2 can be ascribed to color processing.

2.5.4.2 Effect of Contrast on Hemispheric Asymmetry

One might argue that stimulus contrast might affect the hemispheric asymmetry found in Experiment 1-2. Stimulus contrast, however, has been shown to benefit either the left hemisphere, right hemisphere processing, or no hemispheric difference depending on the task characteristics (Christman, 1989). No asymmetry was found in Experiment 1-4, where the contrast changed with the luminance. Both luminance and contrast, therefore, does not seem to contribute considerably to the right hemisphere advantage in color detection.

2.5.4.3 Effect of Practice on Visual Field Difference

In Experiment 1-4, no significant hemispheric difference was observed, which shows that the right hemisphere superiority observed in Experiment 1-2 is due to the detection of color. However, there is a possibility that the lack of asymmetry found in Experiment 1-4 might be due to practice effects. Most participants in the present study were assigned to two experiments. Half of the subjects had participated in Experiment 1-2 and the other half had participated in Experiment 1-1. There are general carry-over effects in psychological experiments. And in a visual half-field paradigm, visual field differences sometimes disappear with practice. Therefore, the observation that there was no hemispheric difference in Experiment 1-4 might be due to the practice effect.

This possibility can be examined by making two comparisons. First is the comparison of reaction times between R-R and L-L in the two groups. No significant difference was observed between reaction times in R-R (292±3.4 ms, mean ± SE) and L-L (289±11.3 ms, mean ± SE) in the 6 right-handed subjects who participated in Experiment 1-2 ($t(5)=0.464$, $p = 0.6621$). Similarly, no significant difference was observed between reaction times in R-R (329±14.5 ms, mean ± SE)) and L-L (326±11.3 ms, mean ± SE)) in the 6 right-handed subjects who had not participated in Experiment 1-2 ($t(5)=0.362$, $p = 0.7323$). Second is the comparison of the mean reaction time difference between RR and LL in these two groups. The difference of reaction times between R-R and L-L was 3.8±8.3 ms (mean ± SE) in the 6 subjects who participated in Experiment 1-2, and was 3.7±10.6 ms (mean ± SE) in the 6 subjects who had not participated in Experiment 1-2. No significant difference was observed between the mean differences (t(10)= 0.012, p = 0.9904). These two comparisons rule out the practice effect as an explanation.

2.5.4.4. Effect of Subject Number Size

In Experiment 1-4, no hemispheric asymmetry was observed in the achromatic targets in the 6 or 12 right-handed participants, while clear asymmetry was found in the chromatic targets in Experiment 1-2 (N=10). It seems impossible that the null results in Experiment 1-4 might be ascribed to a small number of subjects because no asymmetry could be observed even in a larger size of subject (N= 24), in comparison to the size of subject in Experiment 1-2 (N= 6 or 10). Consistent with this view, the effect size (Dunlap et al., 1996) for the null results was smaller (d= 0.025) than those were obtained in Experiment 1-2 (d= 0.678, 0.198; N= 6 who participated in both Experiments 1-2 and 1-4, N= 10, respectively). These findings reject the possibility that a relatively small number size of participants is responsible for the null results in Experiment 1-4.

2.6. Experiment 1-5: Hemispheric Asymmetry of Color Discrimination with Verbal Cues in Right-Handed Subjects

2.6.1. Purpose

In the next experiment, we examined the hemispheric asymmetry of color discrimination. Detection and discrimination require different neural processing, thus different group of neurons are involved in the two processes (Schmidt and Lee, 1998).

2.6.2. Methods

2.6.2.1. Participants

Ten right-handed undergraduate students (5 males and 5 females) with normal or corrected-to-normal vision (mean age 23.0 years, SD 1.0) participated in the present experiment. All of these participants were newly-selected from ten groups of eight subjects in the preliminary experiment as in Experiment 1-1.

2.6.2.2. Apparatus

One of three chromatic solid circles with a diameter of 2 deg (red, x = 0.553, y = 0.313, CIE; green, x = 0.279, y = 0.577, CIE; and blue, x = 0.226, y = 0.151, CIE) were presented at 4 deg laterally from the center of the CRT with a uniform gray background of 10 cd/m^2 as in Experiment 1-2. The luminance of the chromatic stimuli was adjusted to the gray background using the flicker-photometry method as described in Experiment 1-2.

2.6.2.3. Procedures

The subjects were required to press a key quickly after they perceived the color that was not told before starting each session. For example, if the designated color was red, then target colors were green and blue. Each block consisted of 15 trials, 5 trials each for 3 conditions (target color was either non-red, non-green, or non-blue) with a randomized inter-trial interval of 20 sec ranging from 15 sec to 30 sec. A total of 6 blocks, 3 blocks for L-L and 3 blocks for R-R, were performed with a quasi-random order. The mean correct response rate was 94.8±1.03 % (±SE).

2.6.3. Results

Figure 15 indicates that the mean discrimination reaction times in the R-R (367.2±21.0 ms) and the L-L conditions (385.6±21.1 ms, mean ± SE). These values are considerably longer as compared to the simple reaction times. And the variability was larger than that in the detection paradigm (Experiment 1-2). In addition, the mean discrimination reaction time was shorter in the R-R than the L-L condition. A statistically significant difference was found between the R-R and the L-L (paired-t(9)=2.718, p<0.05). Individual analysis showed that the left hemispheric superiority in color discrimination was found in 8 of 10 participants (Fig. 16). These findings suggest that right-handed participants have left hemispheric predominance in a color discrimination task with verbal cues, based on the matching task using color naming.

2.6.4. Discussion

As expected, the discrimination reaction time was longer than the simple reaction time. This finding is consistent with a view that a serial processing of signal detection and discrimination, and a view that the discrimination needs more process than the detection of color (Schmidt and Lee, 1998). The present finding that the discrimination reaction time was shorter in the left hemisphere than in the right hemisphere might suggest that the left hemisphere is dominant in color discrimination. However, before we draw a conclusion, we must consider effect of verbal processing in the present discrimination task. It is well-known that the verbal processing is dominant in the left hemisphere (LeDoux et al., 1977; Gazzaniga et al., 1977), although it is also clear that there are complementary specializations of the right hemisphere (Sperry, 1982). In the present experiment, color discrimination seemed to be based on color naming via verbalization of the stimulus. Thus, the present finding that the discrimination reaction time was shorter in the left hemisphere might be associated mainly with language processing in the left hemisphere. This possibility was examined in the following experiment.

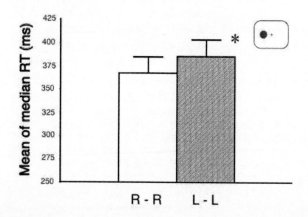

Figure 15. Discrimination reaction times to chromatic stimuli presented either in the right visual field responded by the right hand (R-R) and the left visual field by the left hand (L-L) in 10 right-handed participants. The discrimination task involved verbal cues. The participants were required to press a key if the color was not told before each session (non-matching). Mean reaction time was significantly shorter in R-R than L-L (* $p<0.05$). Mean with SE. Insert shows a schematic sample of stimulus presented in the left visual field.

2.7 Experiment 1-6: Hemispheric Asymmetry of Color Discrimination without Verbal Cues in Right-Handed Subjects

2.7.1. Purpose

In the previous experiment, the left hemispheric superiority in the color discrimination was found. However, in the previous experiment verbal processing was contained in the discrimination task. In this experiment, hemispheric lateralization in color discrimination was examined using a task which does not require verbal processing.

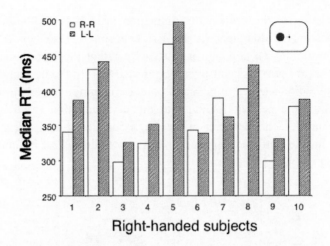

Figure 16. Discrimination reaction times with verbal cues to chromatic stimuli presented either in the right visual field responded by the right hand (R-R) and the left visual field by the left hand (L-L) in each of 10 right-handed participants. In 8 of 10 participants, discrimination reaction time was shorter in R-R than L-L. Insert shows a schematic sample of stimulus presented in the left visual field.

2.7.2. Methods

2.7.2.1 Participants

Eight right-handed undergraduate students (7 males and 1 female) participated in the present experiment (mean age 22.0 years, SD 2.2). All of these participants were newly prepared. They were required to press a key when two stimuli were different in hue or luminance.

2.7.2.2. Apparatus

Two of three chromatic circles (red, x = 0.553, y = 0.313, CIE; green, x = 0.279, y = 0.577, CIE; and blue, x = 0.226, y = 0.151, CIE) or two of three achromatic ones (12, 14 and 18 cd/m^2) were presented at 4 deg lateral to the center of the CRT either in the left or right visual field with a uniform gray background of 10 cd/m^2. The diameters of circles were 2 deg. The chromatic stimuli had the same saturation of 60%. The luminance of the chromatic stimuli was adjusted to gray of 10 cd/m^2 using the flicker-photometry method.

2.7.2.3. Procedures

Participants were required to press a key as fast as possible when the two stimuli presented simultaneously were different either in hue (chromatic stimuli) or luminance (achromatic stimuli). Response was required to be done using the ipsilateral hand to the visual field. Which hand to use was informed before starting each block.

A block consisted of 48 trials; 36 chromatic and 12 achromatic trials with a quasi-random order. Four trials were performed for each condition. For a chromatic trial, one of nine conditions (RR, RG, RB, GR, GG, GB, BR, BG, and BB), and for an achromatic trial, one of three conditions (14-12 cd/m^2, 14-14 cd/m^2, and 14-18 cd/m^2) was tested.

A total of four blocks (discrimination reaction time with R-R or L-L, and simple reaction time with R-R or L-L condition) were carried out for each participant in a quasi-random order. Discrimination reaction times longer than 600 ms and simple reaction time longer than 400 ms were omitted from later analysis. Other procedures were the same as in Experiment 1-2. The data from one subject was omitted from later analysis for achromatic stimuli because the participant made no response to achromatic stimuli in the L-L condition.

2.7.3. Results

Although the discrimination reaction time to chromatic stimuli tended to be shorter in the left hemisphere (386.7±11.2 ms, mean ± SE) than in the right hemisphere (409.6±17.5 ms, mean ± SE), the difference was not statistically significant (paired-t(7)=1.722, p=0.1286) (Fig. 17). Similarly, although a net discrimination time, which was obtained by subtracting simple reaction time from the discrimination reaction time, tended to be shorter in the left hemisphere (R-R: 123.3±10.8 ms, mean ± SE, L-L: 150.8±20.1ms, mean ± SE), no statistically significant difference was found (paired-t(7)=1.867, p=0.1041) (Fig. 18). As for achromatic stimuli, there was no significant difference in discrimination reaction time (R-R: 514.7±10.1 ms, mean ± SE, L-L: 520.4±17.7 ms, mean ± SE, paired-t(6)=0.361, p=0.7303), or even after the net discrimination time was calculated (R-R: 258.3±12.4 ms, mean ± SE, L-L: 273.9±18.7 ms, mean ± SE, paired-t(6)=0.647, p=0.5414). From these findings we could not find any significant hemispheric asymmetry in color discrimination without verbal cues.

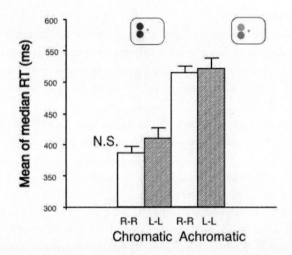

Figure 17. Discrimination reaction times without verbal cues to lateralized chromatic (left) and achromatic stimuli (right) presented either in the right visual field responded by the right hand (R-R) and the left visual field by the left hand (L-L) in 8 right-handed participants. The discrimination task was not dependent on verbal cues. The participants were required to press a key if the two stimuli were different in hue of the chromatic stimuli or in luminance of the achromatic stimuli. There was no significant difference between the reaction times both to chromatic and achromatic stimuli. Mean with SE. Inserts are schematic samples of chromatic (left) and achromatic (right) stimuli presented in the left visual field.

2.7.4. Discussion

Although clear asymmetry was found in the color detection (Experiment 1-2), no hemispheric difference was observed here in the color discrimination reaction time without using language cues. Consistent with this result, Danilova and Mollon (2009) recently reported that there was no asymmetry in color discrimination. However, we should consider a possibility that a longer reaction time has a larger variability. Both in Experiments 5 and 6, discrimination reaction time was longer than simple reaction time. This may easily obscure a subtle difference in reaction time and make it difficult to detect any difference in discrimination reaction time. To elucidate a small but definite difference in reaction times, it is important to adopt some explicit methods and refine current methods to reduce individual variance (Sasaki et al. 2008). Although the net discrimination time showed a slight tendency of shorter reaction time in the left hemisphere (R-R) than right one (L-L) for chromatic stimuli, statistically, no significant difference was found between them. The slight tendency might be due to "different" judgment, because the "different" judgment benefits to the left hemisphere (Magnani et al., 1984). The present findings may suggest that color detection is specialized for the right hemisphere, while color discrimination is not specialized for any hemisphere. Further experiments should be carried out to provide more detailed information about the hemispheric asymmetry in color discrimination.

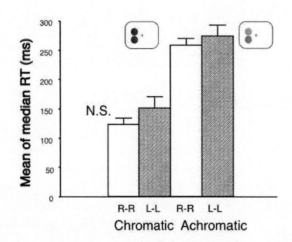

Figure 18. Net discrimination times to stimuli presented either in the right visual field responded by the right hand (R-R) and the left visual field by the left hand (L-L) in 8 right-handed participants. The discrimination task was not dependent on verbal cues. The net discrimination time was calculated by subtracting the simple reaction time from the discrimination reaction time. There was no significant difference between the net discrimination times in the left and right hemispheres both to chromatic and achromatic stimuli. Mean with SE. Inserts are schematic samples of chromatic (left) and achromatic (right) stimuli presented in the left visual field.

It was shown that emotional stimuli are perceived more efficiently by the right hemisphere than by the left hemisphere (McKeever and Dixon, 1981; Smith et al., 2004; Sato and Aoki, 2006). And the right hemisphere plays an important role in producing emotions (Ladavas et al., 1984). The effect of the right amygdala in discriminating emotional faces without primary visual cortices has been suggested (Pegna et al., 2005). A subcortical pathway to the right amygdala may provide a rout for processing unconscious identification of affective expressions in parallel to a cortical route necessary for conscious identification (Morris et al., 1999).

Verbal and non-verbal communication is important for social behaviors in humans. The non-verbal communication includes gestures, eye contact, and expression of emotion, such as disappointment, fear, pleasure, and surprise.

Because the right hemisphere is closely related to emotion, as described above (Ladavas et al., 1984), it is suggested that the right hemisphere plays an important role in the non-verbal communication, by contrast to the verbal communication in the left hemisphere.

Chapter 3

EXPERIMENT 2: PREPULSE INHIBITION OF STARTLE-BLINK RESPONSE USING COLOR PREPULSE

3.1. Background

In the second experiment, contributions of color stimulus to the modulation of the corneal blink reflex were examined in healthy human subjects.

3.1.1. Startle Response

A sudden intense stimulus induces a startle response in many species of animal (Landis and Hunt, 1939). Startle response is one of defensive reflexes to protect oneself from harmful or noxious stimuli (Davis, 1984).

In human studies, the eye-blink reflex was usually recorded as the startle response (Graham, 1975; Lipp and Siddle, 1998). The blink reflex elicited by a corneal stimulation is a component of the startle response, as well as the acoustic startle-blink reflex (Krauter, 1987; Flaten and Elden, 1999) and the electrically-elicited blink reflex (Rossi et al., 1995; Miwa et al., 1998). A relatively weak trigeminal stimulus evokes electromyographic (EMG) activities in the olbicularis occili muscles, while an intense stimulus elicits EMG activities in the other muscles such as the masseter and sternocleidomastoid muscles, in addition to the olbicularis occili. The former is the blink reflex and the latter is termed as the startle response (Valls-Solé et al., 1999).

3.1.2 Prepulse Inhibition

A weak stimulus, which itself does not induce a startle response, presented 30-500 ms prior to a startle stimulus reduces the magnitude of the startle response. This phenomenon is called as prepulse inhibition (PPI, see Hoffman and Ison, 1980), and is widely observed in many animal species including humans (Carlson and Willott, 1996; Swerdlow et al., 1990; Linn and Javitt, 2001; Lipp et al., 1994), except for hamsters (Sasaki et al., 1988, 2007).

PPI is impaired in humans suffering from schizophrenia (Swerdlow et al., 1994) or Huntington's disease (Swerdlow et al., 1995). Impairment of PPI is also observed in rats after mesolimbic dopamine receptors activation (Hoffmann and Donovan, 1994; Caine et al., 1995; Ralph et al., 1999), and in mice lacking the metabotrophic glutamate receptors types 1 and 5 (mGluR1 and mGluR5) (Brody et al., 2003, 2004), which provides an important cue to study the mechanisms for these psychiatric disorders.

Neural circuits of PPI have been widely documented using auditory startle responses in rats. It has been assumed that the PPI occurs at the pontine reticulo-spinal neurons (the caudal pontine nucleus, PnC, see Koch, 1999). However, it is still open about the pathway from where the visual prepulse reaches its effect on the PnC neurons. The superior colliculus has several descending projections to the brain stem nuclei (Redgrave et al. 1987; Dean et al. 1989), including the pedunculopontine tegmental nucleus (PPTg) (Steiniger et al., 1992), an important nucleus of the PPI-mediating circuit. Fendt et al. (1994) showed that PPI decreased significantly, although not completely, after fiber-sparing lesions of the superior colliculus by injections of quinolinic acid bilaterally into the colliculus, suggesting that the descending pathway from the superior colliculus to the brain stem is the main pathway which provides the inhibitory inputs to the PnC. On the other hand, Ison et al. (1991) showed the lack of visual PPI after decortications by using bilateral application of KCl in rats. More recently, bilateral entorhinal cortical lesions reduced PPI in rats (Goto et al., 2002). These findings suggest a possibility that the cortical areas may critically participate in the mechanism of PPI.

3.2. Purpose

It is well-established that color information is preferentially processed in the inferior occipito-temporal visual areas, especially around the fusiform gyrus (Zeki et al., 1991; Corbetta et al., 1991). However, functional roles of color in behavior are not well determined. The purpose of the present study is to examine the modulatory effect of color on the sensorimotor gating. If a differential effect of PPI is obtained for different color prepulses, then the cortical areas may contribute to the PPI mechanism and the color information can exert modulating influences to the sensorimotor gating.

3.3. Methods

3.3.1. Participants

Twenty undergraduate students (18 male and 2 female) with normal or corrected-to-normal vision (mean age 21.9 years, SD 3.1) participated in the present experiment. All participants provided informed consent and were assigned randomly to one of four groups consisting of five individuals.

Each participant received two different chromatic stimuli and one achromatic stimulus as the prepulse; Group R-G (red and green), Group G-Y (green and yellow), Group Y-B (yellow and blue), and Group B-R (blue and red). The achromatic prepulse was common for all of these experimental groups. For example, a participant in Group R-B received red, blue, and the achromatic prepulse, in a quasi-random order.

This experimental paradigm was adopted in order to reduce a total experimental time, which is useful for preventing a decrease of PPI within an experimental session and is good for robustness of the results (Quednow et al., 2006).

The record of one participant from Group G-Y was discarded prior to analysis due to insufficient blink amplitudes, especially on the later trials. A personal report after the experiment showed that this participant was drowsy during the experimental session.

3.3.2. Apparatus

The participant was seated in an isolated, dim experimental room with an ambient illumination level of 0.5 lx, facing to a CRT display (Panasonic TX-D7P35-J, resolution 800 x 600 dots at 60 Hz, 9300K) placed at a distance of 57 cm from the participant's eye. The participant's head was loosely restrained by using a chin rest, and the participant was asked to fixate at a small cross (0.5 deg, 0.5 deg) presented at the center of the CRT display. The background illumination level of the CRT display was the same as the ambient level (Fig. 19).

3.3.3 Prepulse

Four chromatic stimuli (red, 0.553, 0.313, CIE; green, 0.334, 0.531, CIE; blue, 0.230, 0.147, CIE; and yellow, 0.456, 0.410, CIE) and one achromatic stimulus (0.283, 0.320, CIE) were used as the visual prepulses. The main wavelength of these chromatic stimuli was 635 nm (red), 548 nm (green), 463 nm (blue), or 580 nm (yellow), respectively. All of these chromatic stimuli had the same saturation of 60%. The luminance of the chromatic stimuli was adjusted to be equal to 10 cd/m^2 of gray in each participant, by the flicker-photometry method. And the luminance of the achromatic stimulus was 10 cd/m^2. The shape of the visual prepulse was a square and the size of the stimulus was 10 deg x 10 deg in the visual angle. It was presented at the center of the CRT display for 20 ms (Fig. 20). These visual stimuli were generated by a graphic generator (VSG Series Three, Cambridge Research Systems Ltd.), which was controlled by a computer (Power Macintosh 7300/180, Apple) through a serial port via a serial-parallel interface, using a hand-made program (HyperCard, Apple).

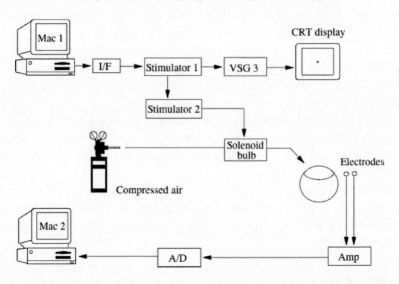

Figure 19. A schematic illustration of the experimental set-up for the prepulse inhibition in humans. Presentation of a visual prepulse and a startle stimulus (a puff of air to the corneal surface) was controlled by a computer (Mac 1) via the interface unit (I/F). The visual stimuli were generated by a graphic generator (VSG 3) and were presented on a CRT display. The lead interval between the pulse and the prepulse was controlled by two stimulators, as well as the duration of pulse and prepulse. EOG signals were amplified (Amp) and stored in another computer (Mac 2) after digitized (A/D) at 400 Hz.

3.3.4 Startle Stimulus

A 50-ms air puff (0.2 MPa, a flow of 2 l/min) directed to the cornea of the left eye was used as a startle stimulus. Distance between the top of a nozzle, which was attached at the end of the air-way, and the surface of the cornea was about 5 cm. Delivery of the air puff was controlled by a solenoid bulb (AB31-02-3-H3A, DC-48V, CKD, Nagoya, Japan) which was placed at the midway of the air-way from the compressed air source and the nozzle. The opening of the bulb was controlled by a combination of two stimulators (SEN-1101 and SEN-3201, Nihon

Kohden). The lead interval between the prepulse and the delivery of the air puff was 100 ms (Fig. 20). This lead interval was chosen because the most sufficient PPI was obtained in a preliminary experiment using the achromatic prepulse ranging from 50-200 ms intervals.

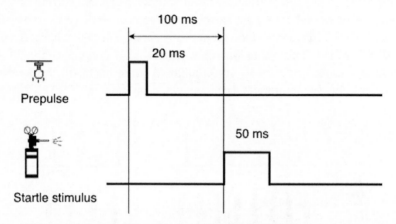

Figure 20. A schematic illustration of the time relations in a prepulse trial. Startle-blink responses were elicited by an air-puff to the corneal surface (0.2 MP, 2 l/min, for 50 ms duration). One of four chromatic stimuli (red, green, yellow or blue, matched to gray of 10 cd/m^2 by flicker photometry, with saturation of 60 %) or an achromatic stimulus of 10 cd/m^2 was used as the prepulse for 20 ms duration. The lead interval of the prepulse and the startle stimulus was fixed at 100 ms.

3.3.5. Recordings of Blinking

A difference in the electrical potentials between the cornea and the retina caused by eye and/or eyelid movements during blinking was detected in the EOG records (Collewijn et al., 1985; Stern and Dunham, 1990;Veltman and Gaillard, 1996; Kong and Wilson, 1998). Two Ag-AgCl surface electrodes with a diameter of 5 mm, placed 1 cm lateral and 1 cm below the lateral edge of the left eye, were used to record the EOG. The signals from these electrodes were differentially-recorded with a ground electrode attached on the forehead (Fpz). The signal was amplified (EEG-4217, Nihon Kohden) with a low-pass filter at 60 Hz, and with a low-cut filter at 0.5 Hz (time constant of 0.3 sec). The EOG recordings lasted for 1 sec in each trial, from 100 ms before and 900 ms after the onset of the startle stimulus and was digitized at 400 Hz (MacLab, A/D Instruments), then stored on a hard disk of a computer (Macintosh Centris 660AV, Apple).

3.3.6. Procedures

In each group, 5 participants received a total of 45 trials with a mean inter-trial interval of 15 sec, ranging from 10 to 20 sec. Only the startle stimulus was presented in the first 5 trials for habituation. Following the habituation trials, the participant received 40 test trials, with or without the prepulse (Fig. 21). Four different groups received different pairs of the prepulse. Three types of prepulse—one gray and two different color prepulses—were presented with a fixed lead interval of 100 ms. This value was chosen because a dominant inhibition was observed at this lead interval in our preliminary experiment. Each participant's behavior was always monitored by a video-camera system.

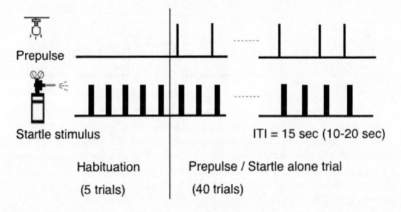

Figure 21. A schematic drawing of experimental procedure for the prepulse inhibition. An experimental session was consisted of 45 trials with a mean inter-trial interval of 15 sec (10-20 sec). In the first five trials, only the startle stimulus was presented as control trials. In the following 40 trials, the startle stimulus was presented with or without the prepulse.

3.4. Results

3.4.1. Measurements of the Response Amplitude

The EOG recordings of the corneal blink response elicited by the air-puff were composed of two positive deflections with a latency at 80 ms and 150 ms, respectively, followed by a large negative deflection at 300 ms (Fig. 22). The early positive deflection was sharp and small in amplitude as compared to the second positive deflection. The early component consisted of high frequency activities, presumably EMG activities of the orbicularis occuli muscles. A peak-to-peak amplitude of the second positive and the large negative components was measured for the amplitude of the startle response.

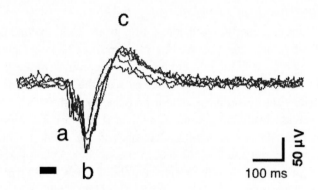

Figure 22. A typical waveform of corneal blink response elicited by an air-puff to the corneal surface recorded by the EOG. Five recordings were superimposed from 100 ms before and 900 ms after the onset of the air-puff. The thick horizontal bar indicates duration of the air-puff for 50 ms. A waveform of the blink response consisted of two positive deflections (a and b) and a large negative one (c). A peak-to-peak amplitude (b-c) was measured as the startle amplitude.

Figure 23 shows a typical example of blink responses in one session (Group R-B). A total of 45 trials were displayed in a line. Although a slight decrement in the blink amplitude was noted during the habituation trials, relatively consistent amplitudes were recorded throughout the session. In most trials without preceding prepulse (marked by filled circles), a clear blink response was elicited by the air puff. On the contrary, a remarkable decrease in the amplitude was observed in the prepulse trials (marked by open circles) as compared to the non-prepulse trials.

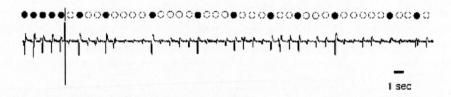

1 sec

Figure 23 . A typical sequence of the startle blink responses consisting of 45 trials in an experimental session of Group R-B. Each trial was sampled for a 1-sec epoch. Open circles indicate trials with the prepulse, and filled circles indicate trials without prepulse. Vertical line indicates end of the habituation period consisting of the first 5 trials. Red, blue and the achromatic prepulses are not distinguished here. Amplitudes of the blink responses markedly decreased in the prepulse trials as compared to those in the pulse alone trials, especially during the early trials.

3.4.2. Typical Example of PPI of the Blink Response

Figure 24 shows superimposed traces of 5 trials each, excluding the first 5 trials. A filled circle indicates the onset of the air puff and an open circle indicates the onset of the prepulse. The left column shows recordings in the early half and the right column shows ones in the later half of the session. The five traces marked 7-24 show the recordings without prepulse from the 7th to 24th trials. A remarkable decrease in the amplitude was found in the following prepulse trials (6-12, 13-18, and 19-25). A similar decrease of the blink amplitude in the prepulse trials was noticed in the later half of the session. As compared to the five trials without prepulse (29-44th trials), the blink amplitude was smaller in prepulse trials either in the 26th-32nd, 33rd-38th, or 39th-45th trials.

3.4.3. Responses to Chromatic and Achromatic Prepulses

The effect of prepulses on the startle amplitudes was examined using % inhibition as an inhibition index, calculated by the following equation:

% inhibition = (mean amplitude in prepulse trials)/(mean amplitude in non-prepulse trials) x 100

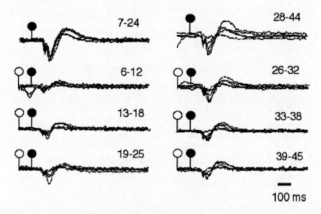

Figure 24 . Inhibition of the startle blink response by the chromatic prepulse in the same session as in Fig. 23. Each group of traces is superimposition of 5 recordings for 1-sec period, from 100 ms prior and to 900 ms after the onset of the air-puff. The open circle and the filled circle indicate the onsets of the prepulse and the air-puff, respectively. Numbers at the right of the traces indicate a rage of trial numbers, from which the recordings were collected. The left column is an early half and the right column is a later half of the session. Startle amplitude decreased in the prepulse trials, both in the early and the later half of the session.

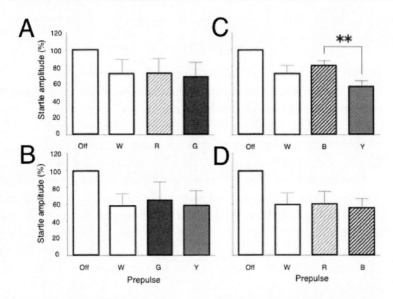

Figure 25. Effect of color prepulse on the amplitude of the startle blink response. Mean blink amplitudes with SE in the chromatic and the achromatic prepulse trials in the four groups; Group R-G (A), Group G-Y (B), Group Y-B (C), and Group B-R (D). Each chromatic prepulse, as well as the achromatic one, significantly decreased the blink amplitude (p<0.05, in all groups). In addition, significant decrease in the amplitude was observed between blue and yellow prepulses (** p<0.01).

Figure 25 shows the effect of the chromatic and achromatic prepulses on the startle-blink responses in the four groups. Control amplitude (Off) was the mean amplitude in the non-prepulse trials, excluding the first 5 trials for habituation. All of the chromatic and achromatic prepulses inhibited the startle amplitude in every group (Fisher's PLSD, p<0.05). In addition, there was a difference in the effect of chromatic prepulses on the startle responses. Significant difference was found between decrease of the amplitude by the blue and the yellow prepulses in Group G-Y (Fisher's PLSD, p<0.01).

3.5. Discussions

3.5.1. Three Types of Blink Reflexes

Blink reflex is essential to protect the eye against corneal drying and damage (Magladery and Teasdall, 1961; Evinger et al., 2002). Blinking is classified into three types according to its motor aspect: spontaneous, voluntary, and reflexive blinking (Bour et al., 2000). The reflexive blinking can be elicited by at least three different types of stimulation in humans.

1) A glabella tap (Pearce, 2008), or electrical stimulation of the supraorbital branch of the trigeminal nerve, elicits EMG responses in the orbicularis oculi muscle, and evokes the blink reflex. The electrically-elicited blink reflex recorded from the orbicularis oculi muscle consists of three components: the two principal ones, R1 and R2, and a third component, R3 (Esteban, 1999). Kugelberg, in 1952, recorded the early-latency R1 and the late-latency R2 EMG responses from the orbicularis oculi muscle (Pearce, 2008). Cruccu et al. (1986) examined the relation of R2 and the corneal reflex, which was elicited by electrical stimulation of the corneal mucosa, in normal subjects and found some different behaviors in habituation and the recovery cycle. The corneal reflex habituated significantly to repetitive stimulations at 0.2–1 Hz but was more resistant than the late component of the blink reflex (R2). In addition, the corneal reflex was less affected by the double schock. From these results they suggest that the corneal reflex is relayed through fewer intramedullary synapses than R2.

2) An intense auditory or visual stimulus evokes the blink reflex. A light flash stimulation evokes the photic early and late responses (Mukuno et al., 1983), and the photic responses were impaired by bilateral occipital lobe lesions (Mukuno et al., 1983). Auditory stimulus also evokes a blink reflex, which is usually considered as the most representative and consistent response of the startle response in humans (Valls-Solé et al., 1999). It was suggested that the physiological characteristics and a brainstem circuitry of the auditory blink reflex may be different from those of the auditory startle response (Valls-Solé et al., 1999). Auditory blink reflexes were considered when auditory stimuli induced responses limited to the orbicularis oculi muscle and auditory startle responses were considered when the responses were induced in other muscles, such as the masseter and sternocleidomastoid muscles (Valls-Solé et al., 1999).

3) A reflex contraction of the human orbicularis oculi muscles can be evoked also by stimulation of the cornea ("corneal reflex") (Fig. 26). The corneal reflex can be elicited by a light mechanical touch to the cornea and the response is bilateral blinking (Ongerboer de Visser, 1980). Mechanical touch and an air-puff to the cornea have been used to produce the corneal reflex (Mukuno et al., 1983, Celebisoy et al., 2000; VanderWerf et al., 2007).

3.5.2. Eyelid and Eye Movements During Blinking

During blinking, both eyelid and eye movements occur. Eyelid movement during blinking is mainly mediated by the levator palpebrae superioris and orbicularis oculi muscles (Evinger et al., 1991; Schmidtke and Buttner-Ennever, 1992; Esteban et al., 2004). The inhibition of the electrical activity of the levator palpebrae superioris muscle precedes and outlasts the reciprocal contraction of the orbicularis oculi (Björk and Kugelberg, 1953). During blinking, stereotypical eye movements occur. In normal human subjects, the eyeball rotates from a straight-ahead position to a nasally-downward one, then followed by a laterally-upward movement during blinking (Evinger et al., 1984; Bour et al., 2000; Collewijn et al., 1985; Riggs et al., 1987; see VanderWerf et al., 2007). These eye movements during blinking have been termed as Bell's phenomenon. However, Bell's phenomenon did not occur during short blinks (Collewijn et al., 1985). On the other hand, the lid closing over the eye causes a difference in the corneal-retinal potential that is evident in the EOG (Stern and Dunham, 1990). Therefore, the EOG can be used for recordings of blinking (Veltman and Gaillard, 1996; Kong and Wilson, 1998).

The neuronal mechanisms initiating the eyelid and eye movement during blinking are not well understood. Recently, however, new evidence was obtained showing that specific areas in the lateral medullar reticular formation are involved in the eyelid and eye movements during blinking (Smit et al., 2005, 2006).

Neural circuits for the blink reflex elicited by the electrical stimulation of the supraorbital nerve have been reported. The trigeminal afferent limb reaches the facial efferent limb by means of a long and complex pathway located at the brainstem bulbopontine level (Esteban, 1999). The corneal reflex circuit has three components: (1) primary cornea afferents; (2) second order trigeminal complex neurons; and (3) orbicularis oculi motoneurons (Henriquez and Evinger, 2007) (Fig. 26).

3.5.3. Neural Circuit for PPI

It has been suggested that the visual prepulse exerts an inhibitory influence to the auditory-startle response at the Pnc via the superior colliculus and PPTg (Koch, 1999). In the case where the auditory prepulse is concerned, an additional pathway from the inferior colliculus to the superior colliculus is involved (Fendt et al., 2001). The auditory evoked potentials that can be recorded in the PPTg with a latency of 13 ms in rats (Ebert and Ostwald, 1991). Although the effective lead interval between prepulse and the startle stimulus depends upon the intensity of prepulse, it ranged about from 20 ms to 500 ms in rats (Hoffman and Searle, 1965) and from 30 ms to 500 ms in human eyeblink response (Graham, 1975).

These facts mean that the subcortical PPI mediating pathway from the superior colliculus to the Pnc via the PPTg play an important role in PPI at a relatively short lead interval (Fendt et al., 2001). PPI at a longer lead interval should be mediated by other neural circuits with more synaptic connections. Consistent with this suggestion, PPI decrement after bilateral lesions of the superior colliculus was not complete but some residual PPI still remained (Fendt et al., 1994).

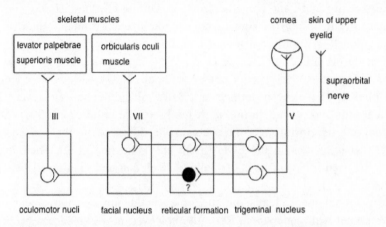

Figure 26. Schematic drawings of neural pathways underlying the corneal reflex. A mechanical stimulus applied to the surface of the cornea or the skin of the upper eyelid elicits action potentials in the trigeminal nerve. They are transmitted to the facial neuron through multisynaptic relays in the reticular formation and elicit contraction of the orbicularis occuli muscles. At the same time, inhibition of the oculomotor neuron, probably via inhibitory interneurons located in the reticular formation, elicits relaxation of the levator palpebrae superior muscles. These responses in the skeletal muscles cause the eyelid closure. III: oculomotor nerve, V: trigeminal nerve, VII: facial nerve.

3.5.4. Effect of Change in Luminance

In the present experiment, visual prepulse was presented on the gray background of the ambient illumination level. Thus, the appearance of the prepulse on the CRT display was accompanied by the change in luminance, as well as the change in chroma. The presentation of the achromatic stimulus elicited only the luminance change, while the presentation of the chromatic stimuli elicited both changes in the luminance and the chroma. The effect of the chroma itself as the prepulse seems to be weak as compared to the luminance because the amount of the inhibition caused by the chromatic prepulse was similar to that elicited by the achromatic prepulse of 10 cd/m^2 (Fig. 25). In addition, in our preliminary experiment using the chromatic stimuli that produced only change in the chroma without accompanying change in the luminance, no significant PPI was observed. However, these findings do not necessarily imply that the luminance is always more effective than the chroma because it has been shown that the effect of the PPI depends on the intensity of the prepulse (Reijmers and Peeters, 1994; Blumenthal, 1996), and because the intensity of the chromatic and the achromatic prepulses were not changed systematically in the present experiment. Moreover, in the present results, there was the significant difference in the effect of inhibition between chromatic stimuli. The startle amplitude was more inhibited by the yellow prepulse than the blue one. These findings suggest that not only the luminance, but also the hue was importantly involved in the PPI.

3.5.5. Cortical Contributions to PPI

It is well known that the color information is processed in the visual cortices around the fusiform cortex (Corbetta et al., 1991; Zeki et al., 1991). Therefore, the present findings suggest that the visual cortex is involved in the visual PPI, at least in human startle responses elicited by the corneal stimuli. It has been suggested that the ventral stream of visual information from the striate cortex to the fusiform cortex is responsible for the processing of color, as compared to the dorsal stream, which engages in the processing of positional cues of the stimulus (Rozenzweig et al., 1999). The ventral stream of the visual information will transmit to the amygdala via the inferotemporal cortex. The neurons in the amygdala project to the PPTg through the accumbens and the ventral pallidum (Koch, 1999). These indirect projections may exert an inhibitory influence on the PPTg. Consistent with this view, it was reported that the central nucleus of the amygdala modulates blink reflex sensitivity in the rabbit (Whalen and Kapp, 1991). Results of several lesion studies are also in line with the view described here. Lesions of the inferotemporal cortex caused severe impairments in the PPI. Reduced PPI with bilateral entorhinal cortical lesions by injections of the ibotenic acid has been reported in rats (Goto et al., 2002). Additionally, the quinolinic acid lesions of the basolateral amygdala significantly reduced PPI without significantly changing startle amplitude (Wana and Swerdlow, 1996). Moreover, blockade of the dopamine receptors in the basolateral amygdala disrupted PPI in a dose-depended manner in the rat (Stevenson and Gratton, 2004). Furthermore, it has been suggested that the medial prefrontal cortex is involved in the PPI circuit (Koch, 1999). Therefore, it is possible for the visual prepulse to reach the PPTg via these cortical areas. Although the precise neural circuit for the PPI of the human corneal reflex is still remained to be determined, the present findings suggest that the visual cortex is critically involved in the human PPI, using the visual prepulse.

Chapter 4

PARALLEL PROCESSING IN THE VISUAL SYSTEM

4.1. Two Visual Pathways

Visual signals starting from the retina are transmitted to the visual cortex via two different pathways; one is the geniculostriate pathway and the other is the extrageniculostriate pathway. The geniculostriate pathway conveys the visual signal to the striate cortex (primary visual cortex, area 17) via the relay cells of the dorsal part of the lateral geniculate nucleus, while the extrageniculostriate pathway conveys the signal to the extrastriate visual cortex (secondary visual cortex, area 18/19) via the neurons in the superior colliculus and the pulvinar nucleus of the thalamus (Fig. 27). The lateral posterior nucleus of the thalamus in rodents is a homology of the pulvinar in monkeys and a homology of the lateral posterior nucleus- pulvinar complex in cats (see Sasaki et al., 2008).

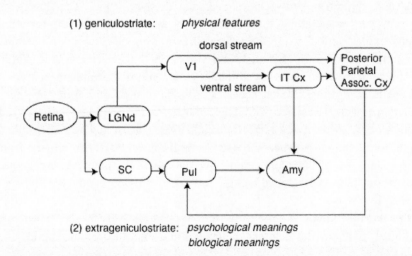

Figure 27. Visual pathways for analysis of physical features and of psychological/ biological meanings of the stimulus. The former is processed by the geniculostriate pathway which branch off into dorsal and ventral streams. These pathways exert modulatory effects on producing emotion at the amygdala (Amy) via direct or indirect top-down pathways. The latter is processed by the extrageniculostriate pathway through the superior colliculus (SC) and the pulvinar nucleus of the thalamus (Pul) to the amygdala. These two systems work in parallel, thus the visual inputs are processed by the dual pathways to the amygdala. LGNd: dorsal part of the lateral geniculate nucleus of the thalamus, V1: primary visual cortex, IT Cx: inferotemporal cortex, Assoc. Cx: association cortex, SC: superior colliculus, Pul: pulvinar nucleus of the thalamus, Amy: amygdala.

Schneider (1969) postulated a separation between the cording of location and identification of a visual stimulus—the retino-tectal and the geniculo-striatal pathways, respectively. The geniculostriate pathway serves for object perception and the extrageniculostriate pathway plays an important role in the visually-guided orientation of eye, head, and body to the stimulus, and in detection of the brightness change (Sasaki et al., 2008). Involvement of the extrageniculostriate system in the processing of the global features of a stimulus, such as brightness, contrast, and intensity, rather than the detailed, local features, which are responsible for the geniculostriate system, has been suggested (Sasaki et al., 2008).

4.2. Two Visual Streams

Two parallel visual streams in the cortex are well known. The cortical flow of visual information starting at the striate cortex diverges into two streams, the dorsal and ventral streams (Ungerleider and Miskin, 1982). The dorsal visual stream is concerned about the processing of spatio-temporal information and visually-guided action, while the ventral stream is involved in the processing of color and object cognition (Goodale and Milner, 1992; Ungerleider et al., 1998).

The geniculostriate pathway in monkeys is composed of magno-, parvo-, and konio-cellular channels; each receives afferent projections from M (magno-cellular, parasol), P (parvo-cellular, midget), and small bistratified retinal ganglion cells, respectively (see Rodieck, 1998). These channels correspond to motion, form, and color processing (see Nicholls et al., 1992; Sincich and Horton, 2005). Extensions of the mago-cellular and parvo-cellular pathways are suggested to be responsible for the dorsal and the ventral streams, respectively (Livingstone and Hübel, 1998).

In cats and rodents, X-type (brta) retinal-ganglion cells project selectively to the dorsal part of the lateral geniculate nucleus, thus contributing to the geniculostriate system, while W-cells (gamma) project to the superior colliculus, which is a part of the extrageniculostriate system. Y-cells (alpha) project both to the lateral geniculate nucleus and the superior colliculus by bifurcating fibers (Hoffmann, 1973; Boycott and Wässle, 1974; Fukuda and Stone, 1974).

X-cells ('sustained' cells) have a relatively small size of receptive field (Peichl and Wässle, 1979), and, thus, the X- system is involved in the analysis of detailed features such as contours of a stimulus, while Y-cells ('transient' cells) have relatively fast conduction velocity (Ikeda and Wright, 1972), and, thus, the Y- system plays a role in the analysis of temporal features such as movements of the stimulus, respectively (see Sasaki et al., 2008). X- and Y- systems correspond to the parvo-cellular and magno-cellular systems in monkeys, respectively (Rodieck et al., 1985), although an debate has been in existence about which cell classes in the monkey are most like that of cat ganglion cell classes (Shapley and Perry, 1986).

The global features of a stimulus are essential for action to the stimulus, and less important for the object perception, which requires more detailed features of the stimulus. Consistent with this view, the extrageniculostriate system contributes to an analysis of global features of a stimulus, and W-cells are mainly involved in the extrageniculostriate system (Sasaki et al., 2008). As compared to the X- and Y-systems, the W-system consists of a heterogeneous group of non-X and non-Y cells. From the evidence that the W-system has relatively slow conduction velocity and relatively low spatial resolution as compared to the X- and Y-systems (Sasaki et al., 2008), it is reasonable to consider that the W-system is an evolutionally-old system. It seems probable that the limbic system, which is also an evolutionally-old brain structure, receives the sensory inputs via the primitive sensory pathway.

It has been shown that there is a heavy projection from the superior colliculus to the pulvinar-lateral posterior complex (cat, Graybiel, 1972; rat, Perry, 1980; hamster, Mooney et al., 1984). Tectal cells, which project to the pulvinar-lateral posterior complex located in the superficial layers of the superior colliculus, are innervated by W-type retinal axons (Hoffmann, 1973; Nagata and Hayashi, 1979). This suggests that W-system may convey visual information to the limbic system.

Table 1 summarizes three systems for a visual signal analysis. Dorsal and ventral streams consist of Y-cell (magno-cellular) and X-cell (parvo-cellular) systems, respectively. The dorsal stream concerns the analysis of spatio-temporal features, while the ventral stream plays an important role in the analysis of figure and color. Thus, the dorsal stream is concerned with information about 'where' (Ungerleider and Miskin, 1982) and vision for 'action' (Goodale, 1993), while the ventral stream is concerned with information about 'what and vision for 'perception. On the other hand, the subcortical pathway from the superior colliculus to the amygdala via the pulvinar nucleus involves W-cells, and is concerned with the analysis of biological meanings (appetitive or aversive) and psychological meanings (pleasant or unpleasant) of the visual signal to produce emotion without acknowledged perceptual awareness.

Table 1. Three pathways for analysis of the visual signal.

pathway	cell type	information	analysis	output
dorsal stream	Y-cell (magno)	where	spatio-temporal (physical) conscious detection => action	
ventral stream	X-cell (parvo)	what	figure & color (physical) conscious detection => perception	
SC-Pul-Amy	W-cell	how	appetitive-aversive (biological) pleasant-unpleasant (psychological) subconscious detection => emotion	

SC: superior collliculus, Pul: pulvinar nucleus, Amy: amygdala

4.3. Three Hierarchies of the Brain

In evolutionally-lower animals such as planarians, adaptive behaviors are controlled by a primitive type of an information-processing mechanism, which is termed as taxis. A planarian is a multi-cellular organism and belongs to the flatworm. It has a very simple nervous system and is one of the primitive animals that has a brain (Agata et al., 1998; Agata, 2008; Aoki et al., 2009). A planarian shows approaching movements to feed such as a block of lever of the chicken (positive chemo taxis) and escaping movements from a bright light (negative photo taxis). The former is necessary to obtain food, and the latter is useful for escaping from predators. Both of these are primitive types of adaptive behavior (Rolls, 1999).

Innate, programmed behaviors in vertebrate consist of reflexive and instinctive behaviors. Many reflexes elicit defensive or appetitive responses to stimuli incoming from outside and thus contribute to our survival. These reflexes are the basis for the conditioned responses in a higher level of adaptive behavior (Pavlov, 1928). The center of the reflex arch is located in the spinal cord or the lower brain stem. More integrated but still automatically-regulated adaptive behaviors such as food-intake, regulation of body temperature, and sexual behaviors are controlled by activities of the hypothalamus, which innervates both the autonomic nervous system and the endocrine system (Fig. 28). Conscious behaviors are closely-related to activities of the cerebral cortex, which developed later in evolution. These stratified behaviors seem to have a close relation to a triune brain model that explains the evolution of the human brain (MacLean, 1970). In this model, the human brain consists of three hierarchies (triune brain) from inside to outside.

4.4. Limbic System

The limbic system is situated deeply inside the human brain, and its corresponding function is a primitive judgment of the incoming stimulus. Whether a stimulus is aversive (dangerous or harmful) or necessary for the organism, it is estimated by the limbic system, especially in the amygdala. As a result of the judgment, a behavioral strategy whether 'approach to' or 'avoid from' the stimulus is determined.

Appetitive and aversive stimuli are well-defined in behavioral studies in animals (Sasaki and Yoshii, 1984; Sasaki et al., 1993). It has been demonstrated that the amygdala is involved in the processing of emotional stimuli (Zald, 2003). Lesion studies have shown that the amygdala is critical for fear and anxiety in rats (Davis, 1992a, 1992b; Falls and Davis, 1995; Malkani and Rosen, 2001). Lesions of the amygdala disrupted fear conditioning measured with fear-potentiated startle in rats (Hitchcock, 1987; Campeau, 1995; Campeau and Davis, 1995). Functional imaging studies showed that the amygdala makes evaluative judgments on appetitive and aversive stimuli (LaBar et al., 1998; Büchel et al., 1998; Sabatinelli et al., 2005). Thus, it is suggested that the amygdala processes knowledge about stimuli and plays a crucial role in processing affective information conveyed by sensory stimuli (Adolphs, 1999; Sander et al., 2003; Williams et al., 2004).

A scale for judgment to an incoming stimulus is ranged from danger, noxious, aversive, dislike to likelihood, appetitive, affective, and needs. This scale is not fixed but flexible in a certain range, and it depends on the drive level of the organism. For example, food can be very attracting objects for a hungry animal, but is neutral for a saturated animal. If the stimulus is noxious or aversive, avoidance behavior will take place, and, at the same time, negative emotions will be produced automatically and unconsciously. If the stimulus is attractive, approaching behavior and positive emotion will be induced.

Aversive stimulus induces a negative emotion at the amygdala and elicits the autonomic and endocrine responses at the hypothalamus to prepare for danger and to alert the incoming danger (Fig. 28).

These primitive types of adaptive responses are performed subcortically without consciousness, and the consequence of the responses will be perceived and interpreted at the level of cerebral cortex. This pattern is very similar for a case of somatic reflex to a noxious stimulus. Spinal reflexes control withdrawal of hand or foot to a noxious stimulus. The ascending sensory information is transmitted to the cortex, and then a series of events that occurred are perceived later.

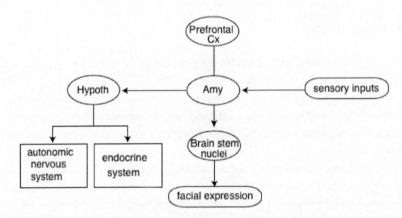

Figure 28. Sensory inputs to the amygdala (Amy) are transmitted to at least two different structures. Aversive or appetitive values are transferred to the hypothalamus (Hypoth) for homeostatic regulation by the autonomic nervous system and the endocrine system. The emotional consequences are expressed outside as a facial expression via the brain stem nuclei, such as the facial nucleus. The activity of the amygdala interacts with those in the prefrontal cortex (prefrontal Cx).

4.5. Dual-Processing Circuits of Visual Inputs

Visual signals are processed not only in the visual system, but also in the limbic system, which is non-specific to the visual processing. The amygdala is the core center for analyzing biological meanings of the stimulus in order to judge whether a stimulus is positive or negative for the organism (Klüver and Bucy, 1939; Rolls, 1999).

Visual informations to the amygdala are conveyed through either the inferotemporal visual cortex or the posterior thalamic nuclei (Fig. 27). Visual pathways to the amygdala have been well-documented in rats. Substantial projections to the amygdala from the lateral posterior thalamic nucleus were found by several retrograde tract-tracing techniques (Doron and Ledoux, 1999). In addition, injections of anterograde tracer biotinylated dextran amine into the lateral posterior thalamic nucleus resulted in heavy labeling in two amygdala-fugal cortical areas: the temporal cortex area 2 and the dorsal perirhinal cortex, and moderate labeling in the lateral amygdaloid nucleus (Shi and Davis, 2001).

A visual stimulus can be transmitted to the amygdala in rats via either geniculocortical (dorsal part of the lateral geniculate nucleus -> primary visual cortex, secondary visual cortex -> temporal cortex area 2 /perirhinal cortex) or extrageniculocortical (lateral posterior thalamic nucleus -> secondary visual cortex, temporal cortex area 2 /perirhinal cortex) pathways, or direct thalamo-amygdala projections (lateral posterior thalamic nucleus -> lateral amygdaloid nucleus). These visual pathways to the amygdala are suggested to be included in fear-conditioning using a visual cue as the conditioned stimulus (Shi and Davis, 2001).

Projections of the perirhinal cortex to the amygdala have been reported both in rats and monkeys (Shi and Cassell, 1999; McDonald et al., 1999; Suzuki, 1996b). It has long been appreciated that the cortex of the temporal pole in monkeys has interconnections with the amygdala. It has been recognized that the medial portion of the temporal pole (part of the perirhinal cortex) has reciprocal projections to the amygdala (Herzog and Van Hoesen, 1976; Aggleton et al., 1980; Turner et al., 1980; Suzuki, 1996a).

These findings suggest that visual inputs are processed both in the visual cortex for object perception and in the amygdala for analysis of biological meanings. These two processes are carried out in parallel in addition to a serial processing. The former depends on the cortical pathway and the tecto-thalamo-amygdala projections, and the latter depends on the cortical top-down projections via the inferotemporal or the posterior parietal association cortex (Fig. 27). The results of Experiment 2 and the fear-potentiated startle (Sasaki and Hanamoto, 2007) suggest that the top-down signals to the amygdala may play a role in modulation of the startle response and of emotion.

4.6 Synchronous Activity of Inferotemporal Cortex and Amygdala

Sabatinelli et al. (2005) reported corresponding functional imaging activity between the amygdala and the inferotemporal cortex during emotional picture viewing and suggested that the identified correspondence represents a structural covariation of affective meaning of the emotional contents. This data is consistent with a view that the cortical top-down pathway transmits visual signals from the inferotemporal cortex, including the perirhinal cortex, to the amygdala during emotional processing.

The perirhinal cortex in both monkeys and rats is composed of two areas (areas 35 and 36) (Suzuki, 1996b). In monkeys, perirhinal areas 35 and 36 form a band of cortex, situated laterally to the full extent of the rhinal sulcus. On the ventral surface of the brain, the perirhinal cortex includes much of the inferotemporal gyrus (Suzuki, 1996b). Both the dorsal bank cortex (area 36) and the fundus of the rhinal sulcus (area 35) project to the entorhinal cortex and amygdaloid nuclei (Shi and Cassell, 1999). The entorhinal cortex also has significant projections to the amygdala (McDonald and Mascagni, 1997).

4.7. Blindsight and Extrageniculate Visual Pathway

Some human patients with lesions to their primary visual cortex demonstrate residual visual capacity, without conscious perception. The preserved ability to accurately respond to visual inputs has been demonstrated (Weiskrantz, 1996). The phenomenon is referred to as blindsight. A possible mechanism for the blindsight that has been proposed is that a subcortical pathway can detect visual stimulus without the primary visual cortex. A patient is able to discriminate emotional facial expressions presented in his blind hemifield despite an extensive lesion of the corresponding striate cortex (Morris et al., 2001). One proposal is that this residual affective ability depends on a subcortical visual pathway comprising the superior colliculus, posterior thalamus (pulvinar), and amygdala (Morris et al., 1999; Morris et al., 2001; Pegna et al., 2005).

Recently, Goossens et al. (2007) examined the neural correlates of phobic fear by exposing subjects who suffer from arachnophobia to a visual presentation of spiders, using a functional-imaging method. They found that "spider phobics" showed a significantly-increased activation in the amygdala and the pulvinar nucleus of the thalamus. These results support the involvement of an extrageniculostriate pathway in the process of phobic fear.

Pulvinar activation, as well as the amygdala activation, has been observed while viewing fearful expressions (Morris et al., 1999). With brief presentations, a patient with complete unilateral loss of the pulvinar was incapable of recognizing fearful expressions in his contralesional field (Ward et al., 2007). They suggest that fear recognition is mediated by the human medial pulvinar and that the cortex in isolation from the entire pulvinar is incapable of recognizing fearful expressions.

From these findings, we learn that the tecto-pulvinar-amygdala pathway is involved in the recognition of an affective feature of an object. This view is further supported by data showing that dysfunction of the amygdala is critically-related to some affective disorders (Mayberg et al., 1999; Drevets, 2003).

4.8. Amygdala and the Affective Disorders

Functional connections between the limbic structures and the neocortex have long been considered critical to the evolution of emotional behaviors (James, 1884; Papez, 1937; MacLean, 1949; Rolls, 1990; Tucker et al., 1995). The limbic structures seem to be essentially included in affective, or mood, disorders. Neuroimaging studies have identified neurophysiologic abnormalities in the amygdala, as well as the anatomically-related areas of the prefrontal cortex, striatum, and thalamus, in mood disorders (Drevets, 2000, 2003). Dysregulation of the interconnection of limbic-cortical pathways is hypothesized to play a role in the pathogenesis of the affective disorders (Mayberg, 1997; Mayberg et al., 1999). Sensory afferents via the thalamus to the amygdala thus seems to provide a main source of the affection, mood, and emotion.

4.9. Amygdala Regulates the Prefrontal Cortical Activity

The amygdala modulates activity in the prefrontal cortex. The prefrontal cortical neurons reduce their spontaneous activity as a function of a degree of fear. And the prefrontal activity is negatively correlated with the activity of the amygdala (Garcia et al., 1999). They suggested that abnormal amygdala-induced modulation of prefrontal neuronal activity may be involved in certain forms of anxiety disorder. Consistent with this view, altered activity in the amygdala and the prefrontal cortex have been reported in mood disorders. Abnormal elevations of resting cerebral blood flow and glucose metabolism in the amygdala have been reported in familial-pure depressive disorders (Drevets et al., 1992; Drevets, 2000; Drevets, 2001). At the same time, reduction of activity in the prefrontal cortex in depressed subjects suffering from unipolar depression, or in the depressed phase of bipolar disorder, has been reported (Drevets, 2001). In contrast, subjects in the manic phase of bipolar disorder showed higher metabolism in the prefrontal cortex than control subjects (Drevets, 2001). These findings strongly suggest that the amygdala plays an important role in anxiety and fear responses, and the dysfunction of the amygdala is critical for the affective disorders.

4.10. Multimodal Processing for Object Recognition

The amygdala is in receipt of sensory information from many modalities. Direct projections from the medial geniculate body to the amygdala have been shown in rats and cats by using the retrograde axonal transport of horseradish peroxidase and fluorescent substances bisbenzimid and nuclear yellow (Ottersen and Ben-Ari, 1979; Maiskii et al., 1984; Doron and Ledoux, 1999; Russchen, 2004). The amygdala receives afferent projections also from the thalamic taste relay and viscerosensory relay neurons (Turner and Herkenham, 1991).

Object recognition is based on sensory information derived not from a single specific modality, but from multimodal information about the object. Recent studies relating multisensory processing revealed that the recognition of an object is performed not as a result of processing in a single modality, but as a result of integration of various sensory perceptions of different modalities (Shimojo and Shams, 2001; Shams et al., 2004). Indeed, visual perception is altered by other sensory modalities (Shipley, 1964; Walker and Scott, 1981; Welch et al., 1986). Also, some neurons in the visual system show multimodal response characteristics, as well as amygdalar neurons (Schroeder et al., 2004; Rolls, 2004). From these findings, it is suggested that the amygdala is involved in the production of emotional responses based on multimodal sensory information.

All of these facts support the hypothesis that the physical features of a sensory signal (such as spatio-temporal information, figure, and color) are analyzed in the cortex, while the biological features (such as positive or negative, and appetitive or aversive), and also psychological features (such as pleasant or unpleasant, and fear, anxiety, or happiness) are analyzed mainly in the amygdala (Table 1). The visual signals to the amygdala are conveyed via three pathways: the cortico-amygdala pathway through the perirhinal cortex, the cortico-pulvinar-amygdala pathway, and the tecto-pulvinar-amygdala pathway. It seems provable that the former two pathways, via the cortex, are concerned with the conscious perception of an object and the subcortical pathway is involved in unconscious or subconscious perception. These three pathways may contribute to amygdalar recognition of biological and psychological meanings of an incoming stimulus to produce emotional responses.

CONCLUSION

In this chapter, I proposed a new model for visual signal processing. It has been thought that the visual signal is processed in the cortex for perception, and then the information is transferred to the limbic system for recognition. Here I propose a dual-processing model in which the visual signal is conveyed directly to the limbic system via a subcortical pathway, in addition to the cortical pathway. The dual-processing circuits of the stimulus provide a base for an explanation of differentiation, or sprit of emotion, and a logical mind, which is processed without and with consciousness, respectively.

ACKNOWLEDGMENTS

I thank to Dr. Akiko Morimoto, Dr. Akira Nishio, and Ms.Sumie Matsuura for substantial help with RT studies. A part of this research was supported by the Ministry of Education, Culture, Sports, Science, and Technology, Grant-in-Aid for Scientific Research (C), No. 15500136, 2003.

REFERENCES

[1]   Adam, J. J. and Van Veggel, L. M. (1991). Discrete finger response latencies in a simple reaction time task. *Perceptual and Motor Skills, 73*: 863-866.

[2]   Adams, W. J. and Mamassian, P. (2004). The effects of task and saliency on latencies for colour and motion processing. *Proceedings, Biological Science, 271*: 139-146.

[3]   Adolphs, A. (1999). The human amygdala and emotion. *Neuroscientist, 5*: 125-137.

[4]   Agata, K. (2008). Planaria nervous system. *Scholarpedia, 3*: 5558.

[5]   Agata, K., Soejima, Y., Kato K., Kobayashi C., Umesono Y. and Watanabe K. (1998). Structure of the planarian central nervous system. *Zoological Science, 15*: 433-440.

[6]   Aggleton, J. P., Burton, M. J., Passingham, R. E. (1980). Cortical and subcortical afferents to the amygdala of the rhesus monkey (Macaca mulatta). *Brain Research, 190*: 347-368.

[7]   Albert, M. L., Reches, A. and Silverberg, R. J. (1975). Hemianopic colour blindness. *Journal of neurology, neurosurgery, and psychiatry, 38*: 546-549.

[8]   Annett, M. and Annett, J. (1979). Individual differences in right and left reaction time. *British Journal of Psychology, 70*: 393-404.

[9]   Aoki, R., Wake, H., Sasaki, H. and Agata, K. (2009). Recording and spectrum analysis of the planarian electroencephalogram. *Neuroscience, 159*: 908–914.

[10]   Barton, J. J., Press, D. Z., Keenan, J. P. and O'Connor, M. (2002). Lesions of the fusiform face area impair perception of facial configuration in prosopagnosia. *Neurology, 58*: 71-78.

[11]   Berlucchi, G., Heron, W., Hyman, R., Rizzolatti, G. and Umilta, C. (1971). Simple reaction times of ipsilateral and contralateral hand to lateralized visual stimuli. *Brain, 94*: 419-430.

[12]   Berry, L. H. (1990). Effects of hemispheric laterality on color-information processing. *Perceptual and Motor Skills, 71:* 987-993.

[13]   Björk A. and Kugelberg E. (1953). The electrical activity of the muscles of the eye and eyelids in various positions and during movement. *Electroencephalography and Clinical Neurophysiology, 5*: 595-602.

[14]   Blumenthal, T.D. (1996). Inhibition of the human startle response is affected by both prepulse intensity and eliciting stimulus intensity. *Biological Psychology, 44*: 85-104.

[15]   Bour, L. J., Aramideh, M. and Ongerboer De Visser, B. (2000). Neurophysiological aspects of eye and eyelid movements during blinking in humans. *Journal of Neurophysiology, 83*: 166-176.

[16]   Boycott, B. B. and Wässle, H. (1974). The morphological types of ganglion cells of the domestic cat's retina. *The Journal of Physiology, 240*: 397-419.

[17]   Brody, S. A., Conquet, F. and Geyer, M. A. (2003). Disruption of prepulse inhibition in mice lacking mGluR1. *European Journal of Neuroscience, 18*: 3361-3366.

[18]   Brody, S. A., Dulawa, S. C., Conquet, F. and Geyer, M. A. (2004). Assessment of a prepulse inhibition deficit in a mutant mouse lacking mGlu5 receptors. *Molecular Psychiatry, 9*: 35-41.

[19]   Bryden, M. P. *Laterality: Functional asymmetry in the intact brain.* New York: Academic Press; 1982.

[20]   Büchel, C., Morris, J., Dolan, R. J. and Friston, K. J. (1998). Brain systems mediating aversive conditioning: an event-related fMRI study. *Neuron, 20*: 947-957.

[21]   Caine, S. B., Geyer, M. A. and Swerdlow, N. R. (1995). Effects of D-sub-3/D-sub-2 dopamine receptor agonists and antagonists on prepulse inhibition of acoustic startle in the rat. *Neuropsychopharmacology, 12*: 139-145.

[22]   Campeau, S. (1995). Involvement of the central nucleus and basolateral complex of the amygdala in fear conditioning measured with fear-potentiated startle in rats trained concurrently with auditory and visual conditioned stimuli. *Journal of Neuroscience, 15*: 2301-2311.

[23]   Campeau, S. and Davis, M. (1995). Involvement of subcortical and cortical afferents to the lateral nucleus of the amygdala in fear conditioning measured with fear-potentiated startle in rats trained concurrently with auditory and visual conditioned stimuli. *Journal of Neuroscience, 15*: 2312-2327.

[24]   Carlson, S. and Willott, J. F. (1996). The behavioral salience of tones as indicated by prepulse inhibition of the startle response: relationship to hearing loss and central neural plasticity in C57BL/6J mice. *Hearing Research, 99*: 168-175.

[25] Celebisoy, N., Varolgunes, N. and Akyurekli, O. (2000). Corneal reflex and blink reflex changes in thalamic hemorrhage. *Electromyography and clinical Neurophysiology, 40*: 95-102.

[26] Christman, S. (1989). Perceptual characteristics in visual laterality research. *Brain and Cognition,11*: 238-257.

[27] Christman, S. (1990). Effects of luminance and blur on hemispheric asymmetries in temporal integration. *Neuropsychologia, 28*: 361-374.

[28] Collewijn, H., Van der Steen, J. and Steinman, R. M. (1985). Human eye movements associated with blinks and prolonged eyelid closure. *Journal of Neurophysiology, 54*: 11-27.

[29] Conway, M. A., Turk, D. J., Miller, S. L., Logan, J., Nebes, R. D., Meltzer, C. C. and Becker, J. T. (1999). A positron. *Neuroimaging and Memory, 7*: 679-702.

[30] Corballis, P. M. (2003). Visuospatial processing and the right-hemisphere interpreter. *Brain and Cognition, 53*: 171-176.

[31] Corballis, P. M., Funnell, M. G. and Gazzaniga, M. S. (2002). Hemispheric asymmetries for simple visual judgments in the split brain. *Neuropsychology, 40*: 401-410.

[32] Corbetta, M., Miezin, F. M., Dobmeyer, S., Shulman, G. L. and Petersen, S. E. (1991). Selective and divided attention during visual discriminations of shape, color, and speed: functional anatomy by positron emission tomography. *Journal of Neuroscience, 11*: 2383-2402.

[33] Cruccu, G. , Agostino, R., Berardelli, A. and Manfredi, M. (1986). Excitability of the corneal reflex in man. *Neuroscience Letters, 63*: 320-324.

[34] Danilova, M. V. and Mollon, J. D. (2009). The symmetry of visual fields in chromatic discrimination. *Brain and Cognition, 69*: 39-46.

[35] Davidoff, J. (1976). Hemispheric sensitivity differences in the perception of colour. *The Quarterly Journal of Experimental Psychology, 28*: 87-394.

[36] Davis, M. The mammalian startle response. In: Eaton, R. C. (ed.). *Neural mechanisms of startle behavior*. London: Plenum; 1984, pp. 287-351.

[37] Davis, M. (1992a). The role of the amygdala in fear and anxiety. *Annual Review of Neuroscience, 15:* 353-376.

[38] Davis, M. The role of amygdala in condiitoned fear. In: Aggleton, J. (ed.). *The amydgala: Neurobiological aspects of emotion, memory and mental dysfunction*. New York: Wiley-Liss; 1992b; pp. 255-305.

[39] Dean, P., Redgrave, P. and Westby, G. W. M. (1989). Event or emergency? Two response systems in the mammalian superior colliculus. *Trends in Neurosciences, 12:* 137-147.

[40] De Valois, R. L. and De Valois, K. K. (1993). A multi-stage color model. *Vision Research, 33*:1053-1065.

[41] Doron, N. N. and Ledoux, J. E. (1999). Organization of projections to the lateral amygdala from auditory and visual areas of the thalamus in the rat. *Journal of Comparative Neurology, 412*: 383-409.

[42] Drevets, W. C. (2000). Neuroimaging studies of mood disorders. *Biological Psychiatry, 48*: 813-829.

[43] Drevets, W. C. (2001). Neuroimaging and neuropathological studies of depression: implications for the cognitive-emotional features of mood disorders. *Current Opinion in Neurobiology, 11*: 240-249.

[44] Drevets, W. C. (2003). Neuroimaging abnormalities in the amygdala in mood disorders. *Annals of the New York Academy of Sciences, 985*: 420-444.

[45] Drevets, W. C., Videen, T. O., Price, J. L., Preskorn, S. H., Carmichael, S. T. and Raichle, M. E. (1992). A functional anatomical study of unipolar depression. *Journal of Neuroscience, 12*: 3628-3641.

[46] Dunlap, W. P., Cortina, J. M., Vaslow, J. B. and Burke, M. J. (1996). Meta-analysis of   experiments with matched groups or repeated measures designs. *Psychological Methods, 1:* 170-171.

[47] Ebert, U. and Ostwald, J. (1991). The mesencephalic locomotor region is activated during the auditory startle response of the unrestrained rat. *Brain Research, 565*: 209-217.

[48] Esteban, A. (1999). A neurophysiological approach to brainstem reflexes. Blink reflex. *Clinical Neurophysiology, 29:*7-38.

[49] Esteban, A., Traba, A. and Prieto, J. (2004). Eyelid movements in health and disease: the supranuclear impairment of the palpebral motility. *Clinical Neurophysiology, 34*: 3-15.

[50] Evinger, C., Bao, J., Powers, A. S., Kassem, I. S., Schicatano, E. J., Henriquez, V. M. and Peshori, K. R. (2002). Dry eye, blinking, and blepharospasm. *Movement Disorders, 17*: S75-S78.

[51] Evinger, C., Manning, K. A. and Sibony, P. A. (1991). Eyelid movements. Mechanisms and normal data. *Investigative Ophthalmology and Visual Science, 32*: 387-400.

[52] Evinger, C., Shaw, M. D., Peck, C. K., Manning, K. A. and Baker, K. (1984). Blinking and associated eye movements in human, guinea pigs and rabbits. *Journal of Neurophysiology y, 52:* 323-339.

[53] Falls, W. A. and Davis, M. (1995). Lesions of the central nucleus of the amygdala block conditioned excitation, but not conditioned inhibition of

fear as measured with the fear-potentiated startle effect. *Behavioral Neuroscience, 109*: 379-387.

[54] Fendt, M., Koch, M. and Schnitzler, H. U. (1994). Sensorimotor gating deficit after lesions of the superior colliculus. *Neuroreport, 5:* 1725-1728.

[55] Fendt, M., Li, L. and Yeomans, J. S. (2001). Brain stem circuits mediating prepulse inhibition of the startle reflex. *Psychopharmacology, 156*: 216-224.

[56] Flaten, M. A. and Elden, A. (1999). Caffeine and prepulse inhibition of the acoustic startle reflex. *Psychopharmacology, 147*: 322-330.

[57] Foundas, A. L., Corey, D. M., Angeles, V., Bollich, A. M., Crabtree-Hartman, E. and Heilman, K. M. (2003). Atypical cerebral laterality in adults with persistent developmental stuttering. *Neurology, 61:* 1378-1385.

[58] Fukuda, Y. and Stone, J. (1974). Retinal distribution and central projections of Y-, X-, and W-cells of the cat's retina. *Neurophysiology, 37*: 749-772.

[59] Garcia, R., Vouimba, R. M., Baudry, M. and Thompson, R. F. (1999). The amygdala modulates prefrontal cortex activity relative to conditioned fear. *Nature, 402*: 294-296.

[60] Gazzaniga, M. S. and LeDoux, J. E. *The integrated Mind.* New York: Plenum; 1978.

[61] Gazzaniga, M. S., LeDoux, J. E. and Wilson, D. H. (1977). Language, praxis, and the right hemisphere: clues to some mechanisms of consciousness. *Neurology, 27*: 1144-1147.

[62] Goodale, M. A. (1993). Visual pathways supporting perception and action in the primate cerebral cortex. *Current Opinion in Neurobiology, 3*: 578-585.

[63] Goodale, M. A. and Milner, A. D. (1992). Separate visual pathways for perception and action. *Trends in Neurosciences, 15*: 20-25.

[64] Goossens, L., Schruers, K., Peeters, R., Griez, E. and Sunaert, S. (2007). Visual presentation of phobic stimuli: Amygdala activation via an extrageniculostriate pathway? *Psychiatry Research: Neuroimaging, 155:* 113-120.

[65] Goto, K., Ueki, A., Iso, H. and Morita, Y. (2002). Reduced prepulse inhibition in rats with entorhinal cortex lesions. *Behavioural Brain Research, 134*: 201-207.

[66] Graham, F. K. (1975). The more or less startling effects of weak prestimuli. *Psychophysiology, 12*: 238-248.

[67] Graybiel, A. M. (1972). Some extrageniculate visual pathways in the cat. *Investigative Ophthalmology and Visual Science, 11*:322-332.

[68] Hannay, H. J. (1979). Asymmetry in reception and retention of colors. *Brain and Language, 8*: 191-201.

[69] Haxby, J. V., Horwitz, B., Ungerleider, L. G., Maisog, J. M., Pietrini, P. and Grady, C. L. (1994). The functional organization of human extrastriate cortex: a PET-rCBF study of selective attention to faces and locations. *Journal of Neuroscience, 14*: 6336-6353.

[70] Hayes, V. and Halpin, G. (1978). Reaction time of the fingers with responses measured on a typewriter keyboard. *Perceptual and Motor Skills, 47*: 863-867.

[71] Henriquez, V. M. and Evinger, C. (2007). The three-neuron corneal reflex circuit and modulation of second-order corneal responsive neurons. *Experimental Brain Research, 179*: 691-702.

[72] Herzog, A. G. and Van Hoesen, G. W. (1976). Temporal neocortical afferent connections to the amygdala in the rhesus monkey. *Brain Research, 115:* 57-69.

[73] Hitchcock, J. M. (1987). Fear-potentiated startle using an auditory conditioned stimulus: effect of lesions of the amygdala. *Physiology and Behavior, 39*: 403-408.

[74] Hoffman, H. S. and Ison, J .R. (1980). Reflex modification in the domain of startle: 1. Some empirical findings and their implications for how the nervous system processes sensory input. *Psychological Review, 87*: 175-189.

[75] Hoffman, H. S. and Searle, J. L. (1965). Acoustic variables in the modification of startle reaction in the rat. *Journal of Comparative Physiology Psychology, 60*: 53-58.

[76] Hoffmann, D. C. and Donovan, H. (1994). D-sub-1 and D-sub-2 dopamine receptor antagonists reverse prepulse inhibition deficits in an animal model of schizophrenia. *Psychopharmacology, 115*: 447-453.

[77] Hoffmann, K. P. (1973). Conduction velocity in pathways from retina to superior colliculus in the cat: a correlation with receptive- field properties. *Journal of Neurophysiology, 36*: 409-424.

[78] Ikeda, H. and Wright, M. J. (1972). Roceptive field organization of 'sustained' and 'transient' retinal ganglion cells which subserve different functional roles. *The Journal of Physiology, 227*: 769-800.

[79] Ison, J. R., Bowen, G. P. and O'Connor, K. (1991). Reflex modification produced by visual stimuli in the rat following functional decortication. *Psychobiology, 19*: 122-126.

[80] Jack, C. R. Jr., Twomey, C .K., Zinsmeister, A. R., Sharbrough, F. W., Petersen, R. C. and Cascino, G. D. (1989). Anterior temporal lobes and hippocampal formations: normative volumetric measurements from MR images in young adults. *Radiology, 172*: 549-554.

[81] James, W. (1884). What is an emotion? *Mind, 9:* 188-205.

[82] Jaskowski, P. (1982). Dependence of simple motor reaction time on luminance in various adaptation states. *Acta Physiologica Polonica, 33:*163-168.

[83] Kanwisher, N., McDermott, J. and Chun, M. M. (1997). The fusiform face area: a module in human extrastriate cortex specialized for face perception. *Journal of Neuroscience, 17*: 4302-4311.

[84] Khedr, E. M., Hamed, E., Said, A. and Basahi, J. (2002). Handedness and language cerebral lateralization. *European Journal of Applied Physiology, 87*: 469-473.

[85] Kimura, D. (1969). Spatial localization in left and right visual fields. *Canadian Journal of Psychology, 23*: 445-458.

[86] Klüver, H. and Bucy, P. C. (1939). Preliminary analysis of functions of the temporal lobe in monkeys. *Archives of Neurology and Psychiatry, 42*: 979-1000.

[87] Koch, M. (1999). The neurobiology of startle. *Progress in Neurobiology, 59*: 107-128.

[88] Kong, X. and Wilson, G. F. (1998). A new EOG-based eyeblink detection algorithm. *Behavior Research Methods, Instruments and Computers, 30*: 713-719.

[89] Krauter, E. E. (1987). Reflex modification by the human auditory startle blink by antecedent interruption of a visual stimulus. *Perceptual and motor skills, 64*: 727-738.

[90] LaBar, K. S., Gatenby, J. C., Gore, J. C., LeDoux, J. E. and Phelps, E. A. (1998). Human amygdala activation during conditioned fear acquisition and extinction: a mixed-trial fMRI study. *Neuron, 20*: 937-945.

[91] Ladavas, E., Nicoletti, R., Umilta, C. and Rizzolatti, G. (1984). Right hemisphere interference during negative affect: a reaction time study. *Neuropsychologia, 22*: 479-485.

[92] Landis, C. and Hunt, W. *The startle pattern.* New York: Farrar and Rinehart; 1939.

[93] LeDoux, J. E., Wilson, D. H. and Gazzaniga, M. S. (1977). Manipulo-spatial aspects of cerebral lateralization: clues to the origin of lateralization. *Neuropsychologia, 15*: 743-750.

[94] Levy, J. (1969). Possible basis for the evolution of lateral specialization of the human brain. *Nature, 224*: 614-615.

[95] Linn, G. S. and Javitt, D. C. (2001). Phencyclidine (PCP)-induced deficits of prepulse inhibition in monkeys. *Neuroreport, 12*: 117-120.

[96] Lipp, O. V. and Siddle, D. A. T. (1998). The effects of prepulse-blink reflex trial repetition and prepulse change on blink reflex modification at short and long lead intervals. *Biological Psychology, 47:* 45-63.

[97] Lipp, O. V., Arnold, S. L., Siddle, D. A. T. and Dawson, M. E. (1994). The effect of repeated prepulse: Blink reflex trials on blink reflex modulation at short lead intervals. *Biological Psychology, 38*: 19-36.

[98] Lit, A., Young, R. H. and Shaffer, M. (1971). Simple time reaction as function of luminance for various wavelengths. *Perception and Psychophysics, 10*: 397-399.

[99] Livingstone, M. S. and Hübel, D. (1998). Segregation of form, color, movement, and depth: Anatomy, physiology, and perception. *Science, 240:* 740-749.

[100] MacLean, P. D. (1949). Psychosomatic disease and the visceral brain: recent developments bearing on the Papez theory of emotion. *Psychosomatic Medicine, 11*: 338-353.

[101] MacLean, P.D. The triune brain, emotion, and scientific bias. In: Schmitt, F. O. (ed.). *The neurosciences: second study program.* New York: Rockefeller Univ. Press; 1970; pp. 336–349.

[102] Magladery, J. W. and Teasdall, R. D. (1961). Corneal reflexes: an electromyographic study in man. *Archives of Neurology, 5* : 269-274.

[103] Magnani, G., Mazzucchi, A. and Parma, M. (1984). Interhemispheric differences in same versus different judgments upon presentation of complex visual stimuli. *Neuropsychologia, 22*: 527-530.

[104] Maiskii, V. A., Gonchar, Yu. A. and Chepega, E. N. (1984). Neuronal populations in the posterior group of thalamic nuclei projecting to the amygdala and auditory cortex in cats. *Neurophysiology, 16*: 176-185.

[105] Malkani, S. and Rosen, J. B. (2001). N-Methyl-D-aspartate receptor antagonism blocks contextual fear conditioning and differentially regulates early growth response-1 messenger RNA expression in the amygdala: implications for a functional amygdaloid circuit of fear. *Neuroscience, 102*: 853-861.

[106] Malone, D. R. and Hannay, H. J. (1978). Hemispheric dominance and normal color memory. *Neuropsychologia, 16:* 51-59.

[107] Mayberg, H. S. (1997). Limbic-cortical dysregulation: a proposed model of depression. *Journal of Neuropsychiatry and Clinical Neurosciences, 9*: 471-481.

[108] Mayberg, H. S., Liotti, M., Brannan, K. S., McGinnis, S., Mahurin, R. K., Jerabek, P. A., Silva, J. A., Tekell, J. L., Martin, C. C., Lancaster, J. L. and Fox, P. T. (1999). Reciprocal limbic-cortical function and negative mood:

Converging PET findings in depression and normal sadness. *American Journal of Psychiatry, 156*: 675-682.

[109] McDonald, A. J. and Mascagni, F. (1997). Projections of the lateral entorhinal cortex to the amygdala: a Phaseolus vulgaris leucoagglutinin study in the rat. *Neuroscience, 77*: 445-459.

[110] McDonald, A. J., Shammah-Lagnado, S. J., Shi, C. and Davis, M. (1999). Cortical afferents to the extended amygdala. *Annals of the New York Academy of Sciences, 877*: 309-338.

[111] McFie, J., Piercy, M. and Zangwill, O. (1950). Visual-spatial agnosia associated with lesions of the right cerebral hemisphere. *Brain, 73*: 167-190.

[112] McKeever, W. F. and Dixon, M. S. (1981). Right-hemisphere superiority for discriminating memorized from nonmemorized faces: affective imagery, sex, and perceived emotionally effects. *Brain and Language, 12*: 246-260.

[113] Miwa, H., Nohara, C., Hotta, M., Shimo, Y. and Amemiya, K. (1998). Somatosensory-evoked blink response: investigation of the physiological mechanisms. *Brain, 121*: 281-291.

[114] Mooney, R. D., Fish, S. E. and Rhoades, R. W. (1984). Anatomical and functional organization of pathway from superior colliculus to lateral posterior nucleus in hamster. *Journal of Neurophysiology, 51:* 407-431.

[115] Morris, J. S., DeGelder, B., Weiskrantz, L. and Dolan, R. J. (2001). Differential extrageniculostriate and amygdala responses to presentation of emotional faces in a cortically blind field. *Brain, 124*: 1241-1252.

[116] Morris, J. S., Öhman, A. and Dolan, R. J. (1999). A subcortical pathway to the right amygdala mediating "unseen" fear. *Proceedings of the National Academy of Sciences, 96:*1680-1685.

[117] Mukuno, K., Aoki, S., Ishikawa, S., Tachibana, S., Harada, H., Hozumi, G. and Saito, E. (1983). Three types of blink reflex evoked by supraorbital nerve, light flash and corneal stimulations. *Japanese Journal of Ophthalmology, 27*:261-270.

[118] Nagata, T. and Hayashi, Y. (1979). Innervation by W-type retinal ganglion cells of superior colliculus neurons projecting to pulvinar nuclei in cats. *Experientia, 35:* 336-338.

[119] Newton, I. (1672). *Opticks: or a treatise of the reflections inflections and colours of light.* New York: Dover Publications; 1952.

[120] Nicholls, J. G., Martin, A.R. and Wallace, B. G. *From neuron to brain* (third edition) Massachusetts: Sinauer; 1992.

[121] Oldfield, R. C. (1971). The assessment and analysis of handedness: the Edinburgh Invetory. *Neuropsychologia, 9:* 97-113.

[122] Ongerboer de Visser, B.W. (1980). The corneal reflex: electrophysiological and anatomical data in man. *Progress in Neurobiology, 15:* 71-83.

[123] Ottersen, O. P. and Ben-Ari, Y. (1979). Afferent connections to the amygdaloid complex of the rat and cat. I. Projections from the thalamus. *Journal of Comparative Neurology, 187:* 401-424.

[124] Papez, J. W. (1937). A proposed mechanism of emotion. *Archives of Neurology and Psychiatry, 38:* 725-743.

[125] Patel, A. D., Gibson, E., Ratner, J., Besson, M. and Holcomb, P. J. (1998). Processing syntactic relations in language and music: an event-related potential study. *Journal of Cognitive Neuroscience, 10:* 717-733.

[126] Pavlov, I. P. *Lectures on conditioned reflexes: twenty-five years of objective study of the higher nervous activity (behaviour) of animals.* (Translated from the Russian by Gantt, W. H.), London: M. Lawrence; 1928.

[127] Pearce, J. M. (2008). Observations on the blink reflex. *European Neurology, 59*: 221-223.

[128] Pegna, A. J., Khateb, A., Lazeyras, F. and Seghier, M. L. (2005). Discriminating emotional faces without primary visual cortices involves the right amygdala. *Nature Neuroscience, 8*: 24–25.

[129] Peichl, L. and Wässle, H. (1979) Size, scatter and coverage of ganglion cell receptive field centers in the cat. *The Journal of Physiology, 291*: 117-141.

[130] Pennal, B. E. (1977). Human cerebral asymmetry in color discrimination. *Neuropsychologia, 15*: 563-568.

[131] Perry, V. H. (1980). A tectocortical visual pathway in the rat. *Neuroscience,* 5: 915-927.

[132] Poffenberger, A. T. (1912). Reaction time to retinal stimulation with special reference to the time lost in conduction through nerve centres. *Archives of Psychology, 23:* 1-73.

[133] Pujol, J., Deus, J., Losilla, J.M. and Capdevila, A. (1999). Cerebral lateralization of   language in normal left-handed people studied by functional MRI. *Neurology, 52:* 1038-1043.

[134] Quednow, B. B., Kühn, K. U., Beckmann, K., Westheide, J., Maier, W. and Wagner, M. (2006). Attenuation of the prepulse inhibition of the acoustic startle response within and between sessions. *Biological Psychology, 71:* 256-263.

[135] Ralph, R. J., Varty, G. B., Kelly, M. A., Wang, Y. M., Caron, M. G., Rubinstein, M., Grandy, D. K., Low, M. J. and Geyer, M. A. (1999). The dopamine D2, but not D3 or D4, receptor subtype is essential for the disruption of prepulse inhibition produced by amphetamine in mice. *Journal of Neuroscience, 19:* 4627-4633.

[136] Ramachandran, V. S. and Blakeslee, S. *Phantoms in the brain: Probing the mysteries of the human mind*. New York: Morrow; 1998.

[137] Redgrave, P., Mitchell, I. J. and Dean, P. (1987). Descending projections from the superior colliculus in rat: a study using orthograde transport of wheatgerm-agglutinin conjugated horseradish peroxidase. *Experimental Brain Research, 68*:147-167.

[138] Reijmers, L. G. and Peeters, B. W. (1994). Effects of acoustic prepulses on the startle reflex in rats: a parametric analysis. *Brain Research, 661*: 174-180.

[139] Rescorla, R. A. and Wagner, A. R. A theory of Pavlovian conditioning: Variations in the effectiveness of reinforcement and nonreinforcement. In: Black, A. H. and Prokasy, W. F. (eds.). *Classical conditioning II. Current research and theory*. New York: Appleton-Century-Crofts; 1972; pp. 64-99.

[140] Rodieck, R. W. *The First Steps in Seeing*. Massachusetts: Sinauer; 1998.

[141] Rodieck, R. W., Binmoeller, K. F. and Dineen, J. (1985). Parasol and midget ganglion cells of the human retina. *Journal of Comparative Neurology, 233*: 115-132.

[142] Rolls, E. T. (1990). A theory of emotion, and its application to understanding the neural basis of emotion. *Cognition and Emotion, 4:* 161-190.

[143] Rolls, E. T. Multisensory neuronal convergence of taste, somatosensory, visual, olfactory, and auditory inputs. In: Calvert, G. A., Spence, C. and Stein, B. E. (eds.). *The handbook of multisensory processes*. London: Bradford Books (MIT Press); 2004; pp.311-331.

[144] Rolls, E. T. *The brain and emotion*. New York: Oxford University Press; 1999.

[145] Rossi, B, Vista, M., Farnetani, W., Gabrielli, L., Vignocchi, G., Bianchi, F., Berton, F. and Francesconi, W. (1995). Modulation of electrically elicited blink reflex components by visual and acoustic prestimuli in man. *International Journal of Psychophysiology, 20:* 177-187.

[146] Rozenzweig, M. R., Leiman, A. L. and Breedlove, S. M. *Biological Psychology*. Massachusetts: Sinauer; 1999.

[147] Russchen, F. T. (2004). Amygdalopetal projections in the cat. II. Subcortical afferent connections. A study with retrograde tracing techniques. *Journal of Comparative Neurology, 207*: 157-176.

[148] Sabatinelli, D., Bradley, M. M., Fitzsimmons, J. R. and Lang, P. J. (2005). Parallel amygdala and inferotemporal activation reflect emotional intensity and fear relevance. *Neuroimage, 24:* 1265-1270.

[149] Sander, D., Grafman, J. and Zalla, T. (2003). The human amygdala: an evolved system for relevance detection. *Reviews in the Neurosciences, 14*: 303-316.

[150] Sasaki, H. and Hanamoto, A. (2007). Shock sensitization and fear potentiation of auditory startle response in hamsters. *Perceptual and Motor Skills, 105:* 862-871.

[151] Sasaki, H. and Yoshii, N. (1984). Conditioned responses in the visual cortex of dogs. I. During wakefulness. *Electroencephalography and Clinical Neurophysiology, 58:* 438-447.

[152] Sasaki, H., Inoue, T., Iso, H., Fukuda, Y. and Hayashi, Y. (1993). Light-dark discrimination after sciatic nerve transplantation to the sectioned optic nerve in adult hamsters. *Vision Research, 33*: 877-880.

[153] Sasaki, H., Iso, H., Coffey, P., Inoue, T. and Fukuda, Y. (1988). Prepulse facilitation of auditory startle response in hamsters. *Neuroscience Letters, 248*: 117-120.

[154] Sasaki, H., Morimoto, A., Nishio, A. and Matsuura, S. (2007). Right hemisphere specialization for color detection. *Brain and Cognition, 64:* 282–289.

[155] Sasaki, H., Nagata, T. and Inoue, T. Functional role of the extrageniculostriate system in visual perception. In: Nilsson, I. L., Lindberg, W. V. (eds.). *Visual perception: New research.* New York: Nova Science Publishers; 2008; pp. 49-89.

[156] Sato, W. and Aoki, S. (2006). Right hemispheric dominance in processing of unconscious negative emotion. *Brain and Cognition, 62:* 261-266.

[157] Schmidt, R. A. and Lee, T. *Motor control and learning: A behavioral emphasis.* Champaign: Human Kinetics; 1998.

[158] Schmidtke, K. and Buttner-Ennever, J. A. (1992). Nervous control of eyelid function: a review of clinical, experimental and pathological data. *Brain,* 115: 227-247.

[159] Schneider, G. E. (1969). Two visual systems, *Science, 163*: 895-902.

[160] Schroeder, C. E. and Foxe, J. J. Multisensory convergence in early cortical processing. In: Calvert, G. A., Spence, C. and Stein, B. E. (eds.). *The handbook of multisensory processes.* London: Bradford Books (MIT Press); 2004; pp. 295-309.

[161] Scotti, G. and Spinnler, H. (1970). Color imperception in unilateral hemisphere-damaged patients. *Journal of Neurology, Neurosurgery, and Psychiatry, 33*: 22-28.

[162] Sergent, J. (1982). Influence of luminance on hemispheric processing. *Bulletin of the Psychonomic Society, 20*: 221-223.

[163] Sergent, J., Ohta, S. and MacDonald, B. (1992). Functional neuroanatomy of face and object processing. A positron emission tomography study. *Brain, 115*: 15-36.

[164] Shams, L., Kamitani, Y. and Shimojo, S. Modulations of visual perception by sound. In: Calvert, G. A., Spence, C. and Stein, B. E. (eds.). *The Handbook of Multisensory Processes*. London: MIT Press; 2004.

[165] Shapley, R. and Perry, V. H. (1986). Cat and monkey retinal ganglion cells and their visual functional roles. *Trends in Neurosciences, 10*: 229-235.

[166] Shi, C. and Cassell, M. D. (1999). Perirhinal cortex projections to the amygdaloid complex and hippocampal formation in the rat. *Journal of Comparative Neurology, 406*: 299-328.

[167] Shi, C. and Davis, M. (2001). Visual pathways involved in fear conditioning measured with fear-potentiated startle: behavioral and anatomic studies. *Journal of Neuroscience, 21*: 9844- 9855.

[168] Shimojo, S. and Shams, L. (2001). Sensory modalities are not separate modalities: plasticity and interactions. *Current Opinion in Neurobiology, 11*: 505-509.

[169] Shipley, T. (1964). Auditory flutter-driving of visual flicker. *Science, 145*:1328-1330.

[170] Sincich, L.C. and Horton, J.C. (2005). The circuitry of V1 and V2: Integration of color, form, and notion. *Annual Review of Neuroscience, 28:* 303-326.

[171] Smit, A. E., Buisseret, P., Buisseret-Delmas, C., de Zeeuw, C. I., Vander-Werf, F. and Zerari-Mailly, F. (2006). Reticulo-collicular and spino-collicular projections involved in eye and eyelid movements during the blink reflex. *Neuroscience Research, 56:* 363-371.

[172] Smit, A. E., Zerari-Mailly, F., Buisseret, P., Buisseret-Delmas, C. and Vander- Werf, F. (2005). Reticulo-collicular projections: a neuronal tracing study in the rat. *Neuroscience Letters, 380*: 276-279.

[173] Smith, S. D. and Bulman-Fleming, M. B. (2004). A hemispheric asymmetry for the unconscious perception of emotion. *Brain and Cognition, 55*: 452-457.

[174] Smith, S. D., Tays, W. J., Dixon, M. J. and Bulman-Fleming, M. B. (2002). The right hemisphere as an anomaly detector: evidence from visual perception. *Brain and Cognition, 48*: 574-579.

[175] Sperry, R. (1982). Some effects of disconnecting the cerebral hemispheres. *Science, 217*: 1223-1227.

[176] Springer, J, A,, Binder, J. R., Hammeke, T. A., Swanson, S. J., Frost, J. A., Bellgowan, P. S.,   Brewer, C. C., Perry, H. M., Morris, G. L. and Mueller,

W. M. (1999). Language   dominance in neurologically normal and epilepsy subjects: a functional MRI study. *Brain, 122:* 2033-2046.

[177] Steiniger, T. L., Rye, D. B. and Wainer, B. H. (1992). Afferent projections to the cholinergic pedunculopontine tegmental nucleus and adjacent midbrain extrapyramidal area in the albino rat. I. Retrograde tracing studies. *Journal of Comparative Neurology, 321*: 515-543.

[178] Stern, J. A. and Dunham, D. N. The ocular system. In: Cacioppo, J. T. and Tassinary, L. G. (eds.). *Principles of psychophysiology: Physical, social, and inferential elements.* New York: Cambridge University Press; 1990; pp. 513–553.

[179] Stevenson, W. and Gratton, A. (2004). Role of basolateral amygdala dopamine in modulating prepulse inhibition and latent inhibition in the rat. *Psychopharmacology, 176*: 139-145.

[180] Sutherland, N. S. and Mackintosh, N. J. *Mechanisms of animal discrimination learning.* London: Academic Press; 1971.

[181] Suzuki, W. A . (1996a). Neuroanatomy of the monkey entorhlnal, perirhinal and parahlppocampal cortices: organization of corticcrl inputs and interconnections with amygdala and strlatum. *Seminars in Neuroscience, 8:* 3-12.

[182] Suzuki, W. A. (1996b). The anatomy, physiology and functions of the perirhinal cortex. *Curent Opinion in Neurobiology, 6*: 179-186.

[183] Swerdlow, N. R., Braff, D. L., Taaid, N. and Geyer, M. A. (1994). Assessing the validity of an animal model of sensorimotor gating defieits in schizophrenie patients. *Archives of General Psychiatry, 51*: 139-154.

[184] Swerdlow, N. R., Mansbach, R .S., Geyer, M. A., Pulvirenti, L., Koob, G. F. and Braff, D. L. (1990). Amphetamine disruption of prepulse inhibition of acoustic startle is reversed by depletion of mesolimbic dopamine. *Psychopharmacology, 100:* 413-416.

[185] Swerdlow, N. R., Paulsen, J., Braff, D. L., Butters, N., Geyer, M. A. and Swenson, M. R. (1995). Impaired prepulse inhibition of acoustic and tactile startle response in patients with Huntington's disease. *Journal of Neurology, Neurosurgery and Psychiatry, 58*: 192-200.

[186] Szabo, C. A., Xiong, J., Lancaster, J. L., Rainey, L. and Fox, P. (2001). Amygdalar and hippocampal volumetry in control participants: differences regarding handedness. *American Journal of Neuroradiology, 22*: 1342-1345.

[187] Tucker, D. M., Luu, P. and Pribram, K. H. (1995). Social and emotional self-regulation. *Annals of the New York Academy of Sciences, 769*: 213-239.

[188] Turk, D. J., Heatherton, T. F., Kelley, W. M., Funnell, M. G., Gazzaniga, M. S. and Macrae, C. N. (2002). Mike or me? Self-recognition in a split-brain patient. *Nature Neuroscience, 5:* 841-842.

[189] Turner, B. H. and Herkenham, M. (1991). Thalamoamygdaloid projections in the rat: A test of the amygdala's role in sensory processing. *Journal of Comparative Neurology, 313*: 295 -325.

[190] Turner, B. H., Mishkin. M. and Knapp, M. (1980). Organization of the amygdalopetal projections from modality-specific cortical association areas in the monkey. *Journal of Comparative Neurology, 191*: 515-543.

[191] Ungerleider, L. G. and Haxby, J. V. (1994). 'What' and 'where' in the human brain. *Current Opinion in Neurobiology, 1994*, 4:157-165.

[192] Ungerleider, L. G. and Miskin, M. Two cortical visual systems. In: Ingle, D. J., Goodale, M.A. and Mansfield, R. J. W. (eds.). *Analysis of Visual Behavior.* Cambridge: The MIT Press; 1982; pp. 549-586.

[193] Ungerleider, L. G., Courtney, S. M. and Haxby, J. V. (1998). A neural system for human visual working memory. *Proceedings of the National Academy of Sciences, 95*: 883-890.

[194] Valls-Solé, J., Valldeoriola, F., Molinuevo,J.L., Cossu, G. and Nobbe, F. (1999). Prepulse modulation of the startle reaction and the blink reflex in normal human subjects. *Experimental Brain Research, 129*: 49-56.

[195] VanderWerf, F., Reits, D., Smit, A. E. and Metselaar, M. (2007). Blink recovery in patients with Bell's palsy: A neurophysiological and behavioral longitudinal study. *Investigative Ophthalmology and Visual Science, 48:* 203-213.

[196] Veltman, A. and Gaillard, A. W. K. (1996). Physiological indices of workload in a simulated flight task. *Biological Psychology, 42*: 323-342.

[197] von Campenhausen, C. and Schramme, J. (1995). 100 years of Benham's top in colour science. *Perception, 24:* 695-717.

[198] Walker, J. T. and Scott, K. J. (1981). Auditory-visual conflicts in the perceived duration of lights, tones, and gaps. Journal of Experimental Psychology. *Human Perception and Performance, 7:* 1327-1339.

[199] Wana, F-J. and Swerdlow, N. R. (1996). The basolateral amygdala regulates sensorimotor gating of acoustic startle in the rat. *Neuroscience, 76*: 715-724.

[200] Ward, R., Calder,A. J., Parker, M. and Arend, I. (2007). Emotion recognition following human pulvinar damage. *Neuropsychologia, 45*: 1973-1978.

[201] Weiskrantz, L. (1996). Blindsight revisited. *Current Opinion in Neurobiology, 6:* 215-220.

[202] Welch, R. B., Duttenhurt, L. D. and Warren, D. H. (1986). Contributions of audition and vision to temporal rate perception. *Perception and Psychophysics, 39*: 294-300.

[203] Whalen, P. J. and Kapp, B. S. (1991). Contributions of the amygdaloid central nucleus to the modulation of the nictitating membrane reflex in the rabbit. *Behavioral Neuroscience, 105*:141-153.

[204] Williams, M. A., Morris, A. P., McGlone, F., Abbott, D. F. and Mattingley, J.B. (2004). Amygdala responses to fearful and happy facial expression. *Journal of Neuroscience, 24*: 2898-2904.

[205] Zald, D. H. (2003). The human amygdala and the emotional evaluation sensory stimuli. *Brain Research Reviews, 41*: 88-123.

[206] Zangwill, O. Handedness and dominance. In: Money, J. (ed.). *Reading Disabilities*. Baltimore: Johns Hopkins Univ. Press; 1962.

[207] Zeki, S., Watson, J. P. G., Lueck, C. J., Friston, K., Kennard, C. and Frackowiak, R. S. J. (1991). A direct demonstration of functional specialization in human visual cortex. *Journal of Neuroscience, 11*: 641-649.

INDEX

A

abnormalities, 51, 60
acid, 30, 41
acoustic, 29, 58, 61, 66, 67, 70, 71
action potential, 40
activation, 30, 50, 61, 63, 67
adaptation, 63
adult, 68
adults, 61, 62
affective disorder, 51
affective meaning, 49
Ag, 33
age, 5, 10, 14, 16, 21, 24, 31
agnosia, 65
air, ix, 32, 33, 34, 35, 36, 38
algorithm, 63
alpha, 45
amine, 48
amphetamine, 66
amplitude, 6, 34, 35, 36, 37, 41
amygdala, ix, 27, 41, 44, 46, 47, 48, 49, 50,
    51, 52, 57, 58, 59, 60, 61, 62, 63, 64, 65,
    66, 67, 68, 70, 71, 72
analysis of variance, 8
anatomy, 59, 70
animals, 46, 47, 66
ANOVA, 8
antagonism, 64
antagonists, 58, 62

anxiety, 47, 51, 52, 59
anxiety disorder, 51
application, 30, 67
aspartate, 64
assessment, 14, 65
asymmetry, ix, 3, 4, 16, 20, 21, 26, 58
audition, 72
auditory cortex, 64
auditory evoked potentials, 39
auditory stimuli, 38
autonomic nervous system, 47, 48
avoidance, 47
avoidance behavior, 47
awareness, 46
axonal, 52
axons, 45

B

behavior, 30, 34, 46, 47, 59
benefits, 26
Benham's top, 1
bias, 64
bipolar disorder, 51
blepharospasm, 60
blind field, 65
blindness, 57